Medicate Me Again

Judith Zielinski Marshall

H·E·A·L·T·H
PROFESSIONS
INSTITUTE

Health Professions Institute, Modesto, California, 1994

Medicate Me Again
by Judith Zielinski Marshall

Photographs by Paul E. Temple, C.P.P.
Remembrance Photography, Portland, Maine

Published by

Sally C. Pitman
Health Professions Institute
P. O. Box 801
Modesto, CA 95353
Phone 209-551-2112

Printed by
Parks Printing & Lithograph
Modesto, California

ISBN 0-934385-62-9

Last digit is the print number 9 8 7 6 5 4 3 2 1

To

Shirley Valencich Sacco,
who never forgets to remind me
she is younger than I am

Acknowledgments

Sally Pitman, Editor, Publisher, an extraordinarily gifted woman and steadfast friend, and the entire staff and associates of Health Professions Institute, especially Vera Pyle, Linda Campbell, and Lori Sookhoo.

Thanks to Linda J. O'Grady, President of IDS, Inc., of Burlington and Worcester, Massachusetts, for the best job in the world, the best transcription team, and the flextime to teach.

Sister M. Berchmans, S.S.J. (Harper Woods, Michigan) for her great teaching and encouragement and prayers over forty years.

Professor Jerzy Maciuszko (Berea, Ohio), who changed my life by his teaching and enhanced my Polish heritage.

In memory of Emily Lou Alford and her work in the Cleveland Public Library as Department Head and Librarian.

In memory of Professor Joseph Ink, Cleveland State University, History Department.

Foreword

Someone (I don't know who) has said something to the effect that if you have lived a long time, you've seen everything. I have lived a *very* long time and do still remember with affection one special young doctor (they don't grow on every bush) much like the one in "Mrs. Dixon Goes to Harvard." He was a pediatrician. In his discharge summary on a small child (who resisted all the doctor's attempts to examine him) he said, "I finally sat down with him on my lap and we played a while. I found that he thought tickling was fun, and while tickling him, I *was* able to palpate his liver."

Judith Marshall has lived a while and has seen lots. She will live long and will have seen more, and I look forward to her future books—written as no one else can—with great expectations.

Vera Pyle

Introduction

It gives me great pleasure to publish this second collection of Judith Marshall's essays. Since I received her first letter in 1980, I have probably been her greatest fan. She has such a way with words, and there are many memorable lines in these essays. I suppose one of my favorites is, "When I was naive enough to believe that hospitals existed for the welfare of patients, great dinosaurs roamed the earth" ("Doctors 10, Handmaidens 0").

Doctors have always been a favorite target of Judith Marshall, and health information managers or medical record directors run a close second. Why? Because she bumps into them in the workplace at every turn, and the *un*professional practices of *some* of them interfere with her doing her job. But other medical transcriptionists and business owners do not escape her sharp tongue either.

Through biting satire she has taken to task hundreds of abusers of people and language that the shy and spineless among us dared not. Oftentimes and in many ways, she has spoken about us and for all of us, and those of us who know her work best laud her talent and the passion that underlies every speech and essay she writes.

The essays in this collection were often written in response to a specific incident or news event provoking "the wrath of Marshall." Thus, the dates of the original speech or publication in *Perspectives* magazine appear after each essay to help the reader place the essay in context. Two essays, "Cows in the Belfrey" (about the bed-and-breakfast business) and "Lost on the Information Highway," were speeches presented to audiences of business owners and have not been previously published.

Although I have read each essay many times over the years, reading this collection in one sitting is an enthralling experience and one that I will enjoy again and again. The tone of *Medicate Me Again* is different and more serious than the earlier *Medicate Me*. I think most readers will agree that the hope and optimism for the medical transcription profession that are almost palpable in *Medicate Me* have been replaced by a heavy dose of realism and cynicism in *Medicate Me Again*. Life is tough, she takes every opportunity to point out, and there is a cloud in every silver lining.

Yet we can identify with her rage, her tears, and her laughter. She makes us cry, especially in "It's All Right to Laugh." We share her desire for precision in medical language ("If You Don't Know the Words, Just Hum"). When she rails at "pompous twits" (doctors) who don't know how to dictate, we feel the same way. And if you're over forty, you may share her pet peeve for those who call strangers and elders by their first name without permission ("Call Me Madam"). "Why should I get my pantyhouse in a twist over the use of first names in medical reports?" It's a problem throughout the healthcare industry, and no one has made the case for use of last names so eloquently.

And she can take criticism as well as dish it out. When one of her friends told her, "You have a big mouth, Marshall" ("File Under G for Gravy"), she wrote, "I accepted that with my characteristic good-natured aplomb, and went home and beat some carpets."

She's not wishy-washy. No one has ever accused her of understatement, and she *is* guilty of overkill at times. She's no fence-sitter, and readers have no illusions on where she stands on any issue. When she castigates an attorney for giving bad advice to medical transcriptionists ("Killing Fleas with Howitzers"), we are aware that *he* wasn't the one with the big gun—Marshall was!

Medicate Me Again contains some of Judith Marshall's finest writing and is an excellent companion volume to the ever-popular *Medicate Me*.

Sally C. Pitman

Contents

Is Medical Transcription What I DO or What I AM?

Every summer I sit on the sand and ponder the cosmic questions of life, as the water laps my aging toes. Who am I, what am I, what does it all mean, and who cares?

There are drinks in the cooler. When I bought the ice for the beach, I recognized the clerk. "So, Geraldine, you work for the Lil Peach now?"

"No," she snapped, her voice like those little pops in phone static. "This is what I do; it's not what I AM."

Geraldine was hot and tired but I got her drift. I'm a medical transcriptionist. Is it what I do or is it what I am? Just an old-fashioned transcriptionist. The kind who knows how to spell all the OLD diseases: poliomyelitis, syphilis, gonorrhea. The kind that people buttonhole with questions of health. Daily living is, after all, wellness and sickness and in-between, okay-I-guess, fine-I-guess. Saying "Hi" in America means "Hello! How are you?" Once in a while someone really tells you how they are.

A friend or relative steps on my shoelace and says, "Say, Judith, you know that medical stuff. What is this medicine I am taking?"

"I have a rash. What does it mean?"

"The doctor says I have hyper, hyper something. Now what could that be?"

If I had a dollar for every time someone asked if I am a nurse, I could wallpaper the spare room. And have you noticed how disappointed people are when you tell them you're not a nurse?

After I moved to Massachusetts from Ohio, I went to the voter registration office and filled out a computer form. Occupation: Medical Transcriptionist. The gum-chewing clerk gave me a petulant look. "It doesn't fit in the boxes. What else are you besides this very long word? How about Secretary? How about Typist?"

"No, I'm not a typist in the pure sense."

By this time she was out of patience and I was out of control.

"Pure or impure, what shall it be? Do you want to vote in this country or not?"

Yes, I surely did want to vote, so for the government, for the Commonwealth of Massachusetts, for God and the flag. I became a MED SEC. Now I fit in the boxes.

Ten years later the census office in my home town sent us a computer form. Our household is listed as "One retired male, one spayed dog, one neutered dog, one med trans." It took ten long years to move from *med sec* to *med trans* and the dogs get better billing.

Is a *trans* better than a *sec*? The next time I voted, one of the inquisitive election workers asked me what sort of medicine I transport and isn't it nice that women can be anything they want to be, even truck drivers.

January 1988

The God-Doctor
Syndrome

Understanding the language of medicine and having the ability to interpret that language is a hallmark of the medical transcription profession.

Many doctors find it incomprehensible that someone not an M.D. or an R.N. can speak their language. They sometimes resent the intrusion into their secret and mystifying world of arcane goings-on. When my husband had emergency eye surgery, I wasn't there. The surgeon called me at work to explain what happened. As doctors often do when explaining things to lay persons, he raised his voice as if I were deaf. People tend to do this with foreigners as well.

"Well, Mrs. Marshall, think of the eye as a globe and—"

"Let's cut the babytalk, doctor. What happened and tell me in medical terms. The local doctor said he went blind in one eye . . . "

"Are you a nurse?" he bristled.

"No, I'm a medical transcriptionist."

"That's nice. We're always looking for good typists; maybe I can throw some work your way. Now, where was I? Oh, yes, think of the eye as a globe, Mrs. Marshall."

Now that I know who I am, I wonder who doctors are. Are they people, too, or have they become technicians? Have the intelligent, well-educated scholarly sorts given way

ST. PHILIP'S COLLEGE LIBRARY

to the number-chanters, whose reports are speckled with laboratory data and little else?

Why are some doctors so arrogant, so overbearing, so maddeningly patronizing, so insensitive, so macho, so chauvinistic, so brusque? Other people say hello. They say, "Kiss my ring, you peasant."

Why can't they tell the difference between IN and ON, *in* the month of May, *on* September 1. Why do they slur over the words they don't understand and make up words and think no one will know the difference? "The GU exam was normal on this *circumscribed* male." "The lungs were clear to auscultation and *precision*." Yes, the same words over and over again on many different histories and physicals. Yes, these are American doctors.

So how did doctors get their particular highfalutin view of themselves? Was it just the higher income or was it something else?

I know how they got that way. I figured it out. We made them what they are. We waited in their offices for hours, smiling weakly and not even asking what the delay was about. Were they really in surgery? The man is a dermatologist, for heaven's sake. Why does one patient say he has the 10:30 appointment, and four others also say they have the 10:30 appointment?

Doctors' offices are just like the airlines. I call and ask if things are running on time; "oh, yes, of course." I get there and there is a two-hour delay. Peter Gott, a physician I adore, writes about this problem in his book, *No House Calls.* "The doctor keeps people waiting because he is so disorganized that he has overscheduled himself. He is hungry to keep his office filled." I understand Dr. Gott's colleagues do not adore him.

Patients who endure unpleasantness have problems with authority figures. I, however, am free of these problems. Having spent my formative years in the clutches of nuns, right through the first year of college, and having spent four years in a convent school where the road to hell was paved with patent leather shoes and pearls and where I learned Latin the old-fashioned way (through stark terror), I have no problems with authority figures. I learned that the priests were coddled, obeyed, respected, and the center of the whole shebang. I came out of it unscathed. Of course I did. When the pastor of St. Joseph's swings through the bingo hall on Tuesday nights to greet the players, I automatically stand up, duck my head, and chant, "Good evening, Fawtherrrrr."

The same with doctors. I went to work in a hospital at the tender age of 14 and was told that the doctors were to be coddled, obeyed, respected, and were, of course, the center of the whole shebang. "But," I stammered, "I thought the hospitals were for the patients." The kitchen crew laughed about that one for hours, but they forgave my naivete´. I was just a kid.

I poke fun at physicians. I tease them, satirize them, draw grotesque caricatures of them and, in general, talk like a tough little cookie. But when one of those white-coated men or women approaches me, I am mesmerized. I rise and say, "Good morning, Doctor. How would you like your coffee, sir, uh, ma'am?" I become irritatingly deferential and reverential. My body starts shrinking in height and I have to restrain myself from genuflecting. They call me *Judy* and I try, I really try, to call them by their first name. For crying out loud, it is someone 23 years old. But all that comes out is "Doctor."

Let me give you an example of how authority works and the immense power we confer upon doctors. It was the summer of 1976. My brother had come up from the Cape to our premier hospital. He had a beard, shorts, sandals, and a scruffy appearance. It was a hazy, sultry Sunday. Paul also had a fever of 102, intense abdominal pain localized in the right lower quadrant, and intractable vomiting. The genius of an intern who saw him just declared Paul a drug addict and sent him home. I was alone in my apartment when Paul called. "I am dying," he said. "Help me." I ran to his apartment in a cotton shift and bedroom slippers. After looking at him for a minute, I decided his assessment was correct. Some mysterious calm came over me and I called the ER of the same hospital which had so inelegantly tossed him out.

"This is Doctor Green from Children's Hospital. Some idiot just discharged my brother when it is clear to me he has acute appendicitis. What was his white count anyway? Wait until I find out who did this. And make it snappy." The nurse was quick to tell me the count was 19,000 with a left shift. The speed with which she answered indicated that the chart was right by the telephone. It was still there when I got Paul back to the ER. I had to bribe the taxi driver with a twenty because he said he would not take sick people in his taxi. Besides waving the twenty at him, I waved an emesis basin they had given Paul and told him authoritatively I was a doctor. No makeup, hair in rollers, miserable cheap clothing—but this guy believed me.

When we arrived in the emergency room it was as if the waters of the Red Sea were parting for the sister-doctor of the poor sick patient. Thirty minutes later Paul was in the operating room. They even handed me the chart. The intern who had discharged Paul mysteriously disappeared. The medical record, I might add, was also altered, with both "drug addiction" and the doctor's name being whited out.

I waited outside the operating room for a very long time. There was no one in Boston to call. There was no one at home in Cleveland. The thought occurred to me that I couldn't keep up the masquerade as a doctor much longer, especially if the resident started asking questions. I need not have worried. The surgeon came out, wearing wooden clogs and a flowered surgical cap, a soaking wet Esther Williams type just out of the pool.

"It was bad, but your brother is alive and he will recover." I forgot everything except that this man was a genius. He had saved my brother's life and I wanted to throw my arms around his feet and strew his path with roses.

And that's how authority works. It is conferred and it is often misused or misperceived, but as long as doctors can cure and cut and heal and help in a mystical way, we are going to worship them.

Well, maybe a little bit.

May 1988

If You Don't Know the Words, Just Hum

Dot and I were enjoying a summer luncheon of poached salmon and egg sauce, first having slipped into a dry martini. "It was one of those weeks," she sighed. "Either the dictating physicians didn't know what they were saying or the transcriptionists made up words and tried to flim-flam the proofreader."

"Not OUR transcriptionists," I retorted.

"No, of course not," she said, "but that sort of thing gets my gander up."

"Your what? Don't you mean 'dander'?"

"Oh, whatever. Same word, isn't it?"

I thought of that old joke, "Why does a hummingbird hum?" Answer: "Because it doesn't know the words."

Maddening medico-babble can begin with one little word. A doctor was pontificating about leg pains. "They were of unclear etiology and not clearly ischemic, though not clearly not ischemic either." My "gander" rose a bit but I transcribed that verbatim because, frankly, I didn't know what else to do. Lest one think a young resident said that, nay, nay. It was a "Hahvahd" man with a distinguished reputation in one of those fashionable troika practices, Lawton, Crest, and Lipton, or as we call them, Larry, Curley, and Mo. The young women call them Larry, Darryl, and the other Darryl.

Some people say they transcribe everything verbatim because "I give it like I get it." This implies we are dispatchers who relay messages and call taxis without any actual thought process. Humbug! Not transcribing verbatim is the wonder and the headache (although my pain is usually much lower down) of medical transcription.

A brilliant doctor dictated explosively like a skier going out of a chute. In neurosurgery, he was a vocabulary master, but let him stray into another specialty and he wobbled. We covered for him until the case of the *Courvoisier uterus*; that's what he called the incision. Checking *Dorland's* yielded the Couvelaire uterus, named for a Paris obstetrician. It made sense to us, so we changed it. Dr. Brain returned the report and said we were mistaken; the word was Courvoisier: We sent him a photocopy of the dictionary page. He rolled it into a ball and sent it back with his secretary. Somewhere in New England is a discharge summary with a brandied uterus. I know he will go to his grave saying *JOHN* Hopkins University and Julia *CHILDS*.

Another physician recited that the patient had a positive Legitimes sign. I thought, how odd; Sophocles, Aristotle, Euripides I know, but who is this ancient Greek? The lovely doctor was very brave in admitting she didn't know how to pronounce it and said, "Operator, just spell *Legitimes* any way you like." Since the patient suffered electric-like shocks down the back, she must have meant *Lhermitte's sign*. From the record, the patient could have had either cord compression or multiple sclerosis. We typed *Lhermitte's sign*, adding a note about pronunciation. We never heard from the doctor so we hope she approved, but perhaps she thought the matter too humdrum to respond.

But, by golly, being right doesn't always endear us to the dictator or make us respected. A lengthy report from a malpractice insurer dealt with an *anaerobe manometer*. The work was tedious and boring, all about engineering and instrumentation. Something kept nagging at me, page after page. Finally, I recognized that *anaerobe* was incorrect. I looked for *manometer* in *Dorland's* and there was *aneroid manometer*, a device that measures pressure in a system as compared to that of a vacuum. The entire summary was revised to reflect the change from *anaerobe* to *aneroid*. The clerical supervisor of the client telephoned to register protest. We were NEVER to do that again, that if we THOUGHT, we PERCEIVED an ALLEGED error, to INDICATE such on a note, but NEVER tamper with the dictation. So there, Ms. Smarty Pants Marshall.

Sometimes we are embarrassed for our dictators who wander off the mark: the novice who always wants Medical Records to *ascertain* copies of reports, who told us that the patient was complaining of pain as a *rouge* to get narcotic medication; a social worker who consistently worries that the patient will suffer the *stigmata* of admission to the detox unit.

I rather like some of the more colorful dictation. "The patient was stiff as hell." Now that's succinct and descriptive. "The thyroid was out of whack." "The patient was not feeling up to snuff." Condition on discharge: "The patient was hanging in there."

Like a candle, dictation has two ends. Here are some humdingers by transcriptionists: downgoing *panther* (plantar) responses; *non-genetic* medication; pain in the upper *asparagus* (esophagus); diminished sensation in *Apache* distribution (a patchy); *decor* is distant (the cor): *insolent*-dependent diabetes; and *tupelo* orthopnea (two-pillow). And one charming Transylvanian looking for lesions of the *oral fangs* (oropharynx).

When the patient was an eminent professor of poetry and held the Siegal Chair (yes, the doctor spelled it), our protegee, no doubt dreaming of the Cape, typed *seagull chair*.

It took a four-letter word to prick my sanctimonious defenses. A prospective client called and asked if I knew how to transcribe the SOAP system. "Yes," I lied. I can transcribe anything. Lemme at it. I know my stuff. All night long I lay awake wondering what this system was and why didn't I know the word *SOAP*. At 8 a.m. in the doctor's office they showed me what they meant: Subjective, Objective, Assessment, and Plan. It was a humbling experience.

Shortly afterward I visited my therapist to help cope with my obsessive-compulsive fascination with words and my passion, yes, passion, for precision in medical language.

My doctor leaned forward conspiratorially and said, "I understand completely and I agree with you. Where would we be without clarity? So, Judith, get your ducks in a row, clear your decks and do what is appropriate and don't do what is inappropriate. Are you comfortable with that?"

The sound of humming filled the room and I felt a pain beginning in my upper asparagus.

July 1988

Hens' Teeth and Blue Moons

Rosebeth is the sort of woman everyone likes. Her disposition is amiable, her countenance sunny, and she types like crazy. When she finishes her eight hours at the hospital, she goes home, fixes supper for her family, changes her clothes, and goes into a small room off the kitchen and transcribes for a couple of doctors. Every other Saturday she works for a plastic surgeon in his office, where she transcribes his clinic notes and letters. She is paid a modest salary at the hospital plus full benefits. The plastic surgeon pays her an hourly wage and the two doctors pay her by the page. Her annual income is less than $15,000.

Ann works for a medical transcription service. She is paid by the character or stroke count. She has been with her present employer for over five years. Her benefits include sick time, holiday and vacation time computed to equal her average stroke count per day. She takes one week of paid vacation per year. She pays half the costs of the health coverage plan; the employer pays half. There is no pension and no profit sharing.

The pay is relatively low but Ann feels that the flexibility of hours, the proximity to her home, and the camaraderie of the office all combine to make this a nice job. Ann also takes tapes home with her to transcribe at night. It works out to $1.25 per page. That's a lot of typing. But if she has a bad week where her counts are low, or she began a new account, or equipment broke down, she feels she must work nights in order to have the weekly take-home pay the same as in a good week. Her benefit package is poor and her salary is less than $15,000. She rarely works less than 50 hours per week.

Millie works full time at home. The hand that rocks the cradle also operates the transcriber and a new IBM PC. All her clients are doctors. For some she photocopies, for some she uses much canned dictation, for some she makes three trips a week to their office to pick up and deliver. For all, she is Wonder Woman.

One doctor has five different types of stationery. One doctor insists on 12-pitch type. One doctor demands double spacing and exotic formatting. Millie spends 40% of her time on the road with the baby in the carseat. Millie cannot get sick, she cannot take a vacation, her phone rings incessantly, and she must spend half days on Sundays doing paperwork and bookkeeping. She has no benefits and her annual gross income is $12,500. But because of the extraordinary hours she works, this comes to about $3.00 per hour.

Millie is proud of her spouse who "helps" her with the housework, but when pressed, she admitted that he does the grocery shopping once a week but refuses to bother with the coupons she clips. He will also empty the dryer and cut the grass. What a prince.

A friend told me that the law of supply and demand doesn't apply to transcriptionists. If there is an urgent national shortage of MTs, why aren't our three worker bees doing better in the labor market?

Now that I live in the country, I've found that plumbers are as scarce as, well, hens' teeth. When I found one with a phone who wasn't deer hunting or fishing or visiting a sick relative, he quoted a price of $75.00 per hour. I gulped and paid it. There are approximately six certified medical transcriptionists in the state but I don't think they get $75 an hour. The doctors here don't get $75 an hour. But I digress. There is no other profession in the United States where women actually pride themselves on working so hard, so long, for so little. I have met service owners who work a seven-day week, but their daughters are in law school or studying engineering so when they graduate from college they will start at $28,000 per. I never heard a group of men at lunch telling each other how many long hours they work and adding to the load on weekends. But transcriptionists brag about "a little on the side."

Is it some chromosome or hormone that drives many of us to work too hard for too little? Yes, there is immense pride in transcribing a mushmouth. There is prestige in working for a great hospital or for a great doctor. But by the time some of us wake up, we find a small pension or no pension, bent shoulders and squinty eyes, and wondering what we can do to supplement our income at age 65.

Women are sensitive and caring and seem to need to be needed. Rosebeth is particularly proud of her two clients. Millie says her clients can't do without her. She says she doesn't care about benefits since she is married. This does not endear her to her peers who claim she grossly undercharges.

All of these women are highly motivated and skilled, but none of them has ever learned to say no or to really negotiate reasonable charges with management or client. When talking with them, I sensed they felt that women's time is not as important as men's time. Is that why the wait is so long at the gynecologist or the pediatrician? I think it is.

Women need to work SMARTER, not harder. They need to work shorter hours, if indeed work they must, for much more pay. They need to do some basic cost accounting on an abacus, on their fingers and toes, or on a calculator.

Time must be counted not just for transcribing but for the photocopying, the driving of ten miles for a 15-minute tape, the collating and sorting. One must learn the tax laws. Profitability should determine whether or not we lift a finger. The successful people in our industry learned to use an adding machine before they learned anything else. As for giving anything away, especially their time, successful people will tell you—in a blue moon.

January 1989

I've Got the
Yellow Pages Blues

The following is extracted from my lead call folder originating from our large medical transcription ad in the Yellow Pages in the Greater Boston area. (The names have been changed to protect the guilty.)

March 18. Mr. Crass of Acme Technology called. They have five hours of a symposium on ophthalmological refractive surgery from Vegas. "No hurry," he said. I told him he had a very exotic specialty there. He said it was professionally recorded. I said it would be at least 10 cents a line for six inches of 10-pitch type, and from what he had told me, it would cost at least $250 and probably more. He sounded very shocked and said he would check around and let me know.

March 30. Follow-up to secretary of Mr. Crass. She said that my price was too high. Then she conspiratorially whispered that they probably will never have it done or get some secretary in the company to work overtime.

April 3. The Center for Genetic Research called. The secretary has a conference tape recorded by professionals on five cassettes of 90 minutes each. She said other companies quoted hourly rates starting at $20 and as high as $36 per hour. I said the line rate would be at least 12 cents per line and I would have to listen to a sample at their office, as I am not that comfortable with the topic. She will call back.

May 9. Penny Tate, who called herself a consultant to the Harvard Community Health Plan, called. She has a two-day conference coming up in June and wanted a rate quote. She was too vague as to the subject, the number of voices, and length of tape. A nice woman but very naive. I spent a great deal of time with her and gave her the names of the big transcription companies who do not advertise in the Yellow Pages. Maybe they can help her. I don't think I want anything to do with this one.

May 23. A woman identifying herself as Victoria Moskal called and said it was she who called previously as Penny Tate and as secretary for the Center for Genetic Research. She claimed that Mr. Crass from Acme Technology had already had the job done BY HER when he called me and that now he refuses to pay her. He claims there were errors in her transcription. She has a small claims court date set for July 13 and she wants me to give her my "rate sheet" for her to use in court to support her fees being within the realm of the current standard.

I told her I don't have a rate sheet and that if I did, I wouldn't send it to her as she, at best, had toyed with my professional time, and at worst, I had been shat on soundly by the whole troupe in this sorry little play. She called her-self a medical transcriptionist but she had never done any transcription before this job. I tried to be supportive and asked her to let me know what happens in small claims court. I sent membership information to her so that she could see that medical transcriptionists are indeed a profes-sional organization in the allied healthcare field. She gave me her address as a post office box.

June 12. The saga continues. Mr. Crass's secretary from Acme Technology called to ask me for a "rate sheet" to do another set of tapes she called ophthalmology, and without my agreeing to do this, she said she must have this rate sheet in order to create a "purchase order." For a fleeting moment I wanted to start screaming something like, "Aha, the jig is up!" or "The game is afoot no longer!" But I simply declined the job and hung up.

For awhile I was more paranoid than usual and felt duped and used. I am going to get letters that ask me why didn't I recognize the woman's voice, the notorious Victoria Moskal in her multiple roles, but transcriptionists know that women do not have distinctive voices with the same frequency as men. (Of course, Vera Pyle does, but you know what I mean.) Why didn't I smell a rat?

This incident raised more questions than it offers for directions in the future, but for me—marketing dollar for dollar, nothing pays for itself like the Yellow Pages. Most callers do ask a price first and I usually say there are many variables and I do have a $500 per month minimum for medical transcription. But p.r.n. jobs, such as that one set of tapes, usually are a matter of a price quote and a turnaround time. Ranges are offered more to callers than per-line fixed prices.

Business telephone numbers do offer legitimacy, especially to the home worker. In future, I will try to be much less gullible, but probably will continue my own "style" of courteous, forthright answers.

October 1988

My Heart
Belongs to Daddy

Maybe it was because he was a situs inversus. When he was a young man and had a routine x-ray, the doctors would dance around him and he got quite a kick out of it. Then there was the x-ray burn. It left a square the size of a large meatloaf on his back and people would comment on it at the beach. "Say, Ted, what happened to your back?" and he would love to tell them.

It was natural that as I began to learn the terminology and as my father began to acquire the diseases, that we should develop a relationship. He is an unrepentant and relentless sedentary smoker. Playing his violin and cutting the grass are about it. He survives with the help of hundreds of years of Polish genes. He had a carotid endarterectomy, cholecystectomy, coronary artery bypass graft. He can't pronounce any of them but he survived them. He can't remember CABG ("cabbage") so he says "the vegetable operation."

Every Christmas I give him a new *PDR* and he spends many happy hours poring over the tiny print, matching his prescriptions to the pictures. Like Lyndon B. Johnson, he bares his scars readily.

The sociologists call us women in our forties and fifties the Sandwich Generation. We are taking care of not only the children and grandchildren, but helping our aging parents who now survive longer. Our parents need us as a buffer between their needs and fears and illnesses, and their doctors and hospitals, insurance companies, and Medicare. Many believe, as my father does, that all doctors and all hospitals are created equal, and no amount of screaming will convince him otherwise.

Father worries about his health incessantly, even when his friends are all dropping dead around him and HE is doing splendidly. He worries about every skipped beat, every bout of indigestion. Spending an evening with him is like being with Oscar Levant.

He wants a paternalistic doctor, a handpatter, a benevolent dictator. He does not want a partner in healthcare. He does not want responsibility for his body, and he does not want control of it. He wants the doctor to take care of everything.

We took my parents to a tranquil New England inn for Thanksgiving. The host greeted everyone warmly at a cocktail party upon our arrival. I introduced my father.

"What will you have to drink?" asked our host. My father said he wouldn't have anything at all, and glanced sorrowfully at the fireplace.

I pulled him aside. "What do you mean, you can't have anything. Have some lovely wine, have a nice beer. You always enjoy those."

"Well, I want to but I can't."

"What do you mean, you can't?" I sputtered and hustled my father into a corner.

"Well, I just took a pill and I am afraid."

"Afraid? Afraid of WHAT?"

"I'm afraid IT will happen."

"WHAT will happen?"

The answer was, "IT."

I had a frozen smile on my face, as guests listened to this exchange. "Please tell me, Father."

"Well, I will have an explosion in my stomach when the beer meets the pill."

My nervous tic returned and I struggled to remain calm. "Well, Dad, I read the *Boston Globe* obituaries every day— call it a morbid sense of humor, call it relief when someone my age dies—but you are right. At least two days a week someone dies because of an explosion in the stomach caused by taking a pill and having a little drink."

I turned to him and said, "This is what you worry about, but three packs a day of Chesterfields and fourteen cups of coffee you DON'T worry about?"

I got hysterical and had to leave the dining room. My father had a nice beer and enjoyed supper immensely.

March 1989

Note: Thaddeus J. Zielinski died of lung cancer in Cleveland on March 7, 1989, at the age of 75. The last thing his daughter said to him was. "Dad, you have nothing to be afraid of anymore."

Billet-Doux

After months of sitting here transcribing and gazing out at a bleak frozen landscape, I know spring has arrived in the Northeast Kingdom of Vermont. Our giant maple trees sprouted minty-green leaves, a Baltimore oriole is singing, and the swallows are darting about. I can see the cows in the fresh pastures just beyond the church spire, on the perimeter of the village, and the mountains are lush and new again. The afternoon light slants toward my glass of iced tea and it bursts into glowing amber light, as an oboe concerto begins on the CBC. (That's the Canadian Broadcasting Company, not complete blood count.)

Sounds idyllic, doesn't it? The home-based medical transcriptionist creates her own perfect environment, the incredulous blend of technology and glorious nature. The right equipment and lighting, the right references, the right client mix for the right money, and the dream of every true obsessive/compulsive personality—total control. No wardrobe hassles, no subways, no commute, no public bathrooms, no old bag of a supervisor breathing down my neck. Heaven, you say? Well, what's wrong with this picture?

Isolation, my darlings, that's what. All that communication is flowing just like the Barton River—in one direction. When every call is a toll call and the hospitals I work for can be in a different time zone, what chance do I have to speak or write to a physician about his dictation? Any note from me would be scooped up by an overzealous clerk who will shred it or give it a burial at sea. The supervisors twitter that they would never dream of upsetting the doctor.

I am the bee in the surgical mask. I want a surgeon whose words are sharp and decisive and definitive and bold the way his incisions are. I want a dictator whose knowledge of anatomy is precise and rapid and fluent. A crisp, fresh delivery, some humanity of phrasing. ("Condition on discharge: Dead." Oh, please.) Howzabout it, Doc? I want to know that what is happening under those surgical drapes has some meaning for you, or is the only inspiration you get in your chest?

Use the power of your voice. All right, you are no Shadoe Stevens or Sally Kellerman, but vocalize for me. Don't dither. There are surgeons in practice for years who can make a routine cystoscopy sound like a sonata. It's not the vocal cords that make the music, it's the heart strings. There are wonderful dictators who maintain their balance on a precipice of conflicting emotions. They dictate about patients who destroy their lives with drugs and alcohol, or their unborn children, and I hear no scorn or disapproval in their voices. There are good doctors who dictate psychiatric horror stories and never flinch. They never laugh at the patient who eats only red, white, and blue foods.

I can only give the transcription accuracy. They give the dictation integrity. They give the record exactitude. They maintain the patient's dignity. Some old woman dies in an inner city hospital at age 84 with a complex history, and the resident gives it his best shot and dictates that record as if it were going to be preserved under glass in the archives. I like people like that. They are going to be fine doctors.

Perhaps you know some doctors like this. Clip this paragraph and put it in their mailbox. Tell them it reminds you of them and how really great they are and how you ought to know—you sit there eight hours a day, listening. Tell them you see their code on a printout or their name on a log and you can't wait to sit down and transcribe because it is such a pleasure. So he suffers from withdrawal symptoms—he is a Southerner, after all. So she peppers her dictation with non sequiturs like, "This elderly nonagenarian," but she is clear and thorough. And she says "Good morning" and "Thank you." That counts a lot with me.

And for the rest of you pompous twits who parade as the world authorities on quotation marks and semicolons and who devise clever little abbreviations known only to you and God, well, did you think you would make a clean get-away from the wrath of Marshall? There are no hyphens in "soft brown formed stool," adnexa are adnexa, not *adnexae*, and don't say *Eppy* when you mean *epinephrine*. You are a regular puu-puu platter of errors. It is like transcribing Ricky Ricardo and you are not an ESL dictator. I get so tired of listening to you "splain" your convoluted laboratory data. Pertinent positives and negatives, please.

I drop down to my knees and pray to Our Lady of Formatting that once, just once, you will dictate the preoperative and postoperative diagnoses first, not last, in the report. And listen up, dentists. If you want to be called Doctor and wheel around the OR and be a big cheese, follow the same rules as everyone else.

That wouldn't be a bad paragraph to mail to some guilty furball.

As we approach July 1, known as the Doctor Year, or Year of the Earwig if you wear a headset, here are some dictation pointers for you fledgling docs.

1. For heaven's sake, **look at the format**. Give the diagnoses at the beginning of the summary, if that is what your hospital requires. Do not abbreviate diagnoses. Learn about DRGs.

2. **Give us all the information**. You won't save any time in the long run by skipping it and thinking the trolls who live under the bridge in Medical Records can fill it in.

3. **Get organized**. We don't care if you sound like a munchkin; we can wait a few seconds here and there for the precise word. But rattle that chart around and curse about missing EKGs and you will begin your career here as an unloved wretch. (And probably go on to become full professor and head of the department.)

And maybe with your generation, we can forever put an end to the practice of dictating the first words, "And a carbon copy to . . ."

Happy New Year, boys and girls.

May 1989

File Under G
for Gravy

My mailbags are stuffed with letters from women who want to work at home, preferably for themselves, not for a transcription company. Some want to add a client or two in addition to their jobs at the hospital or service. It's the old syndrome in this business. If we can't change the pay scales or the recognition, let's work more hours.

I spent a fascinating ten hours yesterday typing nothing but EEGs (zzzzzzzz) and thinking about what women are running from as much as what they are running to. Rarely articulated, but always simmering beneath the surface, is the yearning to be free from the boundaries of the office.

And the other women in the office.

I tell aspiring self-employeds that it is a myth to consider women as your friends. SOME of them are your friends. Employment problems are not really money or workload, taxes or benefits. The key problem is relationships. A good friend (male) said to me, "You know, you are a great transcriptionist. But you rile people up, you tee them off. You are too outspoken, too demanding, too vocal. You ask questions, you ruffle feathers, stir up the waters. You are the last person I would call to do a p.r.n. transcription job for me. I want someone docile and compliant. You have a big mouth, Marshall."

I accepted that with my characteristic good-natured aplomb, and went home and beat some carpets. Somewhere there is a middle ground between Uriah Heep and Queen Elizabeth I, but I haven't found it. There are some women at work I was pleased to escape from.

The Old Bag (God, am I turning into one?) I despised less for fussiness and being crotchety than for perpetuating ad nauseum the idea of the medical transcriptionist as the handmaiden of medical records. She kissed so many backsides she suffered from bunburn. I worked with the mother of them all in the basement of a large Boston hospital. She looked the part, too. A formidable woman, corseted, sensible shoes, graying hair in a bun pierced with a pencil. A voice like a Valkyrie, hooded eyes behind immaculate glasses, and the fastest red pen in the Northeast. In those days there were no word processors. We retyped what Mrs. Dunstin ordered (Dunstin the Dragon, she was). Want to work at home? The Old Bags are still around and usually the liaison between you and the hospital.

The Perfection Nut (also called the Anal-Retentive medical transcriptionist) is the person who phones doctors all the time to ask picayune questions or buttonholes them in the corridor. She has Life Savers in her desk lined up in neat little rows. Her reference books are filed by color and height and width. She cleans constantly. Alcohol, Windex, Pledge, moist towelettes, dental floss, toothpicks, feather duster. Well, no wonder she produces only six reports a day. But they are perfect reports. And very clean.

Speed Demons are just the opposite. Their work stations are pigpens, visited mainly by fruit flies. Tattered books, sloppy minds, they tend to be aloof from the group. They have talent and agility but no team spirit or interest in their work, very often leaving early and chirping, "Good night, slaves."

But it's the Mother-Wife-Homemaker I run from. First, it is obvious that this woman does not need to work. It is a social function for her. Her husband has a great job and great benefits and we all know it because she won't shut up about it. Her work is adequate and could be better if she were not on the phone constantly, running her home and checking on the children. She is organized enough to call the plumber, arrange for car repair, and order a cake, all on hospital time. When she has a break, she uses it for a break. God forbid she would spend a dime and make a call in the corridor.

Friction often erupts between this woman and the single and the divorced, the mother struggling to raise her children alone. The situation can become incendiary when the Mother-Wife-Homemaker is a part-time worker who spends time catching up socially at the water cooler or floundering around with a new procedure that was implemented on her day off, but she won't read the instructions. This tension is intensified in the office setting of medical transcription with management trying to fill three shifts seven days a week.

As finely groomed as she is, the Mother-Wife-Homemaker does not see herself as a professional. She is marking time, a temporary measure that can last for decades. This is something to occupy the yawning empty spaces of dull afternoons. The money is extra, file under G for Gravy. While we scurry to pay the mortgage, to make the rent, the Mother-Wife-Homemaker is buying a summer home. While we admire her industriousness, we resent hearing so much about it.

The Organizer Chatterbox has too much of a good thing as feminine traits go. Every time we see her she has her hand out for the sunshine fund, the holiday parties, the contribution for the new office plant (the old one died from ammonia fumes emanating from the Perfection Nut's desk). The last thing on my mind for any holiday is to spend it with the same bunch I work with, eating tired canapes that taste like cat food on stale crackers and curtseying to the doctors and administrators who deign to drop in for a paper cup of pineapple punch laced with vodka. Unless the Old Bag made the punch; then there is no vodka.

The labor force is younger and the baby showers explode in number like sand fleas on a hot August day. While I budget for getting my hair dyed, my teeth crowned, my veins stripped, and my arthritis medicated, I am subsidizing the baby boom and buying tiny clothes and rattles. And the perpetual rounds of farewells (just a drink and sandwich at the local pub and a little memento of the wonderful two years at St. Pancreas) nickel and dime me to death.

The truth is, there is no sisterhood, no grand camaraderie of women, no feminist pervasive scheme or humanist scheme for that matter, in the work world. Jealousy, petty infighting, and a distinct lack of cool rationality continue to plague the woman worker.

Successful women don't think with their ovaries. We must learn to disagree on work issues and work styles without personalizing them (although I tend to personalize EVERYTHING; it's part of my charm). Men know how to compartmentalize. They scream at each other, viciously attack each other, use their secretaries to beat each other over the head, then smile and have lunch or play racquetball.

But men are not divided into two groups—those who must work and those who choose to work. Women are. This is the root of many office conflicts.

Computers, overnight mail, fax machines, growing acceptance of the home worker (note, I am not saying *approval*) are combining to change office politics and provide new challenges for managers and home workers alike, especially in medical transcription, our growing multimillion dollar industry.

July 1989

Lighten Up, Ladies

Unless you were in a coma the past few weeks, it would be impossible to ignore the controversy generated by entrepreneur Jeanne Sellers, president of ML&M Services, Inc., The Medical Transcription Company, based in Atlanta. An ad was placed in the *Journal of the American Medical Record Association* (AMRA) in September 1989, depicting a home worker in medical transcription.

And what an ad! Graphic and punchy, this was every medical record director's or doctor's nightmare when they send out a tape to be transcribed. The young woman sits at her computer, her food and cigarettes at the ready, baby screaming in the playpen, food cooking on the stove. The attire is a bathrobe and curlers. But the caption was the corker. The transcriptionist was calling her friend to gossip about a neighbor whose medical record our gal was transcribing. "Madge, you won't believe what I just found out about your neighbor!" The message to the prospective client is that the advertising company does not use home workers, only in-house transcriptionists. They were telling the customer, this is what we do NOT employ.

My first reaction was hysterical laughter. I thought the ad was funny. Then I wondered who the ad agency was since these people created the perfect horror. As the mail

30

piled up and the phone calls came in, I realized that women (I didn't hear from any men about it) were really upset about this ad. They were infuriated, and boy, did they take it personally.

Several issues are operating here: Image and confidentiality sanctimoniously layered with a tired and overworked sense of what constitutes professionalism. What struck me was that so much negative female energy was used to beat Jeanne Sellers to a pulp as if she and her company were in the puppy-drowning business while flying the swastika from their corporate office.

I don't know the woman but it seems to me she is a business executive who took a calculated risk and has a commitment to hiring the best, keeping the work in-house, and training her staff in confidentiality, among other things. She has consistently supported AAMT. She pays taxes on her employees, doesn't slither away into the netherworld of "contractors" and "subcontractors," and she pays a decent wage (yes, I checked). As an executive in a multimillion dollar industry, Ms. Sellers made a marketing decision. Period.

To me, her targets were scores of nefarious racketeers who feed on the homebound woman's problems, who pay field-hand wages, who sweet-talk hospitals and doctors into hiring their firms because, after all, they can charge lower prices. Of course they can. These unscrupulous bums aren't paying their workers overtime, profit-sharing, health insurance, AAMT dues, or encouraging career development. Sellers is. She is battling the jerks who don't want their workers to know about AMRA or AAMT. Rather like keeping women barefoot and pregnant.

Perhaps I paint the glass too darkly. There are perfectly legitimate folks out there doing medical transcription, and while they don't blatantly lie, just try to let a client track a particular report. It's in a garage in Birmingham or a trailer in Montana or an attic in Houston or a basement in Boston.

It's on someone's kitchen table or in their purse or in the car or on the sink. That report may even be in my mountain aerie office. "For God's sake, Judith, if the client knew that this work was in Vermont, they would kill me."

Do women who work at home all wear business suits and makeup, sitting primly at the computer from 9 to 5? Give me a break. Working in my jammies is high on my list of perquisites. Wearing a bathrobe is de rigueur at 2 a.m. around here and that's when a lot of transcription is done. Now that we crisscross the time zones on our high-tech flying carpet, what are office hours? About like hospital hours— never-ending. Unless those hair rollers are picking up Radio Free Europe, so what? Food, coffee, and cigarettes in the work area are likely in a private setting but are not unknown in the hospital or office.

So was all this karma circulating because the woman in the picture was a distracted slob or because she was a blabbermouth? I think more the former. Listen to these excerpts from angry readers who wrote to *JAMRA* and complained loudly enough so that the ad was pulled: "Offended," "insult to self-employed women transcriptionists," "derisive to all women regardless of their occupation," "hurt, disappointment, humiliation and anger," "slapped in the face" ("professional" used eleven times in one brief letter), and going up to "extreme displeasure and embarrassment." Oh, I forgot "infuriating," "absolutely appalled," and "blatant defamation."

One woman wrote to me, "God forbid a doctor should see it." The doctors don't have to see it, my dear. Many of them encourage the hand that rocks the cradle to do their typing. They want those wages low. They want that ten-minute tape turned around overnight. They want it driven those ten miles. No true professional transcriptionist would touch these doctors or their work, with its low-volume, high-aggravation ratio.

Our image is terrible but within every stereotype is a kernel of truth, and the women working at home in a variety of occupations have a way to go from being "cottage industry" to "telecommuters." Housewives still have a terrible image and it spills over into home-based businesses.

We need to educate the consumers (doctors and hospitals) to hire men and women affiliated with AMRA and AAMT. The latter's Code of Ethics, Number 9, states, "Protect the privacy and confidentiality of the individual medical record to avoid disclosure of personally identifiable medical and social information and professional medical judgments." A company or hospital which actively promotes a program of teaching about confidentiality and a clear mandate of what happens (fired on the spot) when it is breached is what I like to see.

Loose lips still sink ships and I'm hoping to keep this barge afloat a while longer. But there are so many *nonmedical* personnel handling my records in today's world, it terrifies me. Who learns what dark secrets is pretty much a crapshoot as far as I'm concerned.

Personally, I am sorry this ad was pulled. I am sorry so many nice women got all riled up and had to rush to their typewriters to tell, basically each other, that they are as professional as heck. I am sorry that so much emotion was involved; hell hath no fury . . .

No, I don't worry about the fate of medical records in the hands of bona fide CMTs and ARTs and RRAs and dedicated personnel. I worry about the thousands of women out there who are a threat to the business/profession art/science of what we do. I worry about the women who have no credentials, no education, no knowledge of business, no library card, and no sense. They write to me and they call me and they want an instant guide to home transcription. They readily admit they have no business plan, no reference books, no IDEA of what they are doing, but they want me to help them get into my profession. And the sad thing is, they probably will.

I can get crazy with emotion too. I just point my self-righteous indignation, like a wobbly windsock, in another direction. I want AMA recognition for medical transcriptionists. That's something worth building up a head of steam for. I want higher pay scales in hospitals, and supervisors who fight like bantam roosters for this instead of knuckling under. I want to see the law of supply and demand work to such a degree that no medical transcriptionist ever has to work two jobs or type "a little on the side" just to *survive*. I want to outlaw the use of the word "girls" in all hospitals and offices.

Pogo was right. We have met the enemy and they is us.

January 1990

Whining and Dining

About five years ago, I wrote a column entitled "Fat Chance" in which I was truly obnoxious, hooting about a spectacular weight loss achievement. I was convinced I would never gain any of it back. Pass the humble pie. As soon as I quit starving and square dancing, it was do-si-do into old bad habits.

All of my recipes were marked, "Serves six, or two if they are Marshalls." If my professional organization charged people like me by the pound, there would be no dues increase. They could add a wing onto their building. But how could someone as smart as me evidently not know how to eat?

LOW FAT DIET AND EXERCISE is the answer to permanent weight control. Why are we spending millions of dollars in the diet industry? I have paid people to starve me, brainwash me, exercise me, puncture me, humiliate me, and weigh and measure me like a piece of pork (they probably thought so, too). And that was just the diet merchants, not the gyms and salons. I bought an exercise bike that tells me my pulse, blood pressure, rate of speed, and even croaks encouragement in a hoarse staccato computer voice—*you can do it, you can do it, you can do it.*

I have done it. I keep doing it. Veterans of fat wars have chomped through it all. Lose 70, put back 50, lose 50, put back 90. If the equation is fat equals stupid, take me to the head of the class. How easy to rationalize that large sizes are okay, but my tired frame with small bones was never meant to carry more than 120 pounds. Once again, in my new environment in the Northeast Kingdom, I searched for thinness.

Overeaters Anonymous was too religious for me, an amorphous cosmic pantheism. The pressure of self-disclosure was too great. In Vermont, where the cows outnumber the people, can anyone be anonymous?

After the OA meeting, a woman turned to me and asked, "What is your name again? I would hate to be telling all this personal stuff to someone I didn't know."

Weight Watchers, it seemed to me, spent all their time shopping for food, weighing, measuring, discussing, eating and counting, filling out forms, and having a whale of a good time. How much money do they spend on gorgeous television commercials to sell food—and does the corporation really care if people lose weight or if people buy their prepackaged food?

My twin devils are time and boredom. The only thing left in my narrow vision was Optifast. And the only thing narrow about me was my vision. An enormous weight loss in three months of fasting, and the team approach (physician, psychologist, and dietitian) were all very appealing. The cost was nearly $3000 and cleverly charged in upside-down pyramid fashion. I lasted five weeks.

Perhaps it was because all the printed material had to bump down to the lowest common denominator of intelligence. The "homework" consisted of such exercises as multiple-choice questions.

You are now in the program and taking only liquids. Your friend encourages you to eat at a party. Your answer should be (select A or B):

A. Please remember I am on a special program and cannot eat foods now but in a few weeks I will be able to eat regular food. In the meantime, I appreciate your support.

B. You really are an insensitive jerk. Leave me alone. I can't eat anything.

I chose the B answer. It was wrong.

The team members were all young and very thin. They were extremely maternalistic with the women and deferential to the men. It was truly difficult not to laugh when they passed out official-looking wallet cards with a red cross symbol, saying that if we fainted with hunger in an airport, we were somehow to produce this card and be revived by three ounces of lean chicken. The silly talk and hardee-har-har joviality were at first annoying, then depressing. One man suggested the first night we all go down to one of those places that serves all you can eat and *pig out,* as he delicately put it, and wouldn't that give the waitresses a fit to see us all coming.

If the others thought fat grams arrived via Western Union or varicella was a pasta, I didn't stick around long enough to know. I was surprised and disgusted by the lemming-like eagerness of the women, and the men as well, to divulge personal details of their lives that God knows were interesting only to them. The various revelations of what passed through their digestive tracts and how it reached its final destination would make a gastroenterologist blush.

The psychologist was young and eager but fell short of the mark on life experience or even group leadership experience, and any deviation from the week's outline caused her great agitation. What we were drinking was always referred to as The Product (reverential tone and genuflection), while I squirmed in my plastic chair and wondered how high the drug company shares were climbing.

Being pent up in that ship of fools was bad enough, but when one fiftyish business executive lyrically discussed his bout of influenza and his consequent hunger and craving for the comfort of a soft-boiled egg, I was ready to bolt. Instead of just eating the damn egg and having some juice and a lie-down, this fellow had been trained so well by the Fatspeak program, he called the office and spoke to a secretary, who told him to drink hot tea. And he did. Like a good little boy.

Folks, I don't know what the answer is. I only know what it isn't. For me. For now. I thought a women's group experience (I had not expected the men) would help us to deal with anger, depression, and self-hatred. I thought we could transcend talk about junk food. I thought we would discuss sexuality and life changes and not just regurgitate what some smart ad executive wrote up in the manual.

I agree with something Barbara Edelstein, M.D., wrote many years ago in *The Woman Doctor's Diet for Women*. "My feeling is that the overweight female responds best to a one-to-one relationship where you can challenge her, refute her without embarrassing her, and compel her to come to grips with herself, her own tricks and evasions."

So what am I eating and what's really eating me? I am nibbling back to the basics. Low fat, low calorie diet, and moderate exercise, for which I will pay no one. Many women volunteered to talk to me about their Optifast (and other) successes. I rejoice with them while mourning my own perceived failure. Perhaps I will find a therapist who does not take my problem lightly. As for my dollars perpetuating the bloated diet industry, well, I am just fed up.

March 1990

Want a Piece of Candy, Little Girl?

Adapted from a luncheon address delivered on May 5, 1990, to medical transcription business executives at the first national conference sponsored by Health Professions Institute in San Francisco.

How on earth can I tell this distinguished audience anything about the origins of the transcription business, I asked myself. Then I thought about my experiences and felt perhaps I can. I was born in Cleveland and worked my way through school. In that town, at that time, for night and weekend work, the choices were factories and hospitals. I chose hospitals.

I worked for the high and the mighty and the great entrepreneurs. I've worked for hospitals and services since the 1950s in Ohio, Kentucky, and Massachusetts. I owned my own company and worked as a solo self-employed and even temped in more than twenty-five hospitals in the greater Boston area.

Since writing for the *Journal of AAMT* for several years and more recently for *Perspectives*, I have received a wealth of mail which provides me a peek at the labor market. These have included "I have a computer and type rather well" and "I don't know anything about medical transcription but I am a court stenographer." And the one from the woman who had many years of experience as a medical secretary. She had just taken a two-year course in medical terminology and told me that she just loved to "transcrip" and what sort of "transcripping machine" did I have, and that she just can't wait to get into the "transcripping business."

Many of you know I am American by birth, Polish by descent, and Scotch by infusion . . . and I am a real '90s woman . . . 40-something. I was around for Pearl Harbor and I was there the day they walked on the moon. I am somewhere between Midol and estrogen. My work history spans carbon paper in 1955 to modems and macros.

And I spent most of the '80s whining. I went to my therapist and whined for hours. "Stop whining," said my doctor. I said, "Look, I PAY you to listen to me. I can't whine to my co-workers or friends anymore." That decade of me, me, me, and what's wrong with my boring work and stupid doctors, has been transformed into something different and something better, thanks to Prima Vera Publications and Health Professions Institute.

Yes, I am a '90s woman. I have an IRA, TV, VCR, CDs, my HEENT is still PERRLA, and my lungs are clear to P&A since I quit smoking. I have an ulcer, and I am in a hotel full of people who all know their cholesterol counts. We have microwaves, touchtone dialing, laptop computers, laser printers, and irons which turn themselves off—for those of us who still iron. My ears are pierced, my hair is dyed (I have been told I look like a maple tree in high season), and I am up to here with oat bran. We drink bottled water and we recycle everything now. Along with many of you, we are waging war on nonbiodegradable plastics. We conserve propane and fuel oil.

We eat no tuna from companies using dolphin-catching nets, and unless that mink died of old age or committed suicide after a tragic love affair, you won't see me in fur. I want to live in a world where only movies are shot, not guns. I know better than to vacation in Beirut or Northern Ireland or South Africa. I don't eat fresh vegetables in the Ukraine or touch reindeer meat in Lapland.

A true Sagittarian, I have taken a bath in Bath, watched gold convoys at Fort Knox, and I have been kissed so hard it wrapped my teeth around my ankles. I have been pinched in the Pitti Palace, climbed the Acropolis, and walked on the Appian Way. I have been jailed in East Berlin and treated for tear gas in my face during an uprising in Poland. I have flirted with buckaroos in Texas and fished with the Indians up in Canada. I have traded rubles in a women's toilet in Moscow.

But there is no thrill like my work. I really love what I do. Transcription in the '50s in a Catholic hospital created a lot of memories. I remember the nuns and the basements and the sacred records, the self-immolation and sense of sacrifice with which we were imbued. I remember the flickering red vigil lights, the portrait of the Sacred Heart, and the clean, waxed slippery floors. There were flowers on all the May altars during the month of the Blessed Mother. I remember, too, Tommy the diener making dates in the morgue with the young girls and trying to talk them into going into the freezer with him.

How did the nuns and the hospital get what they wanted out of the workers? Back then people had a conscience, they had a work ethic and loyalty to the hospital, the church, the school and family. Doing a good job was the norm. It was also here that the God-Doctor Syndrome (a subject about which I often speak) was born.

A few words about doctors. My, my, my, how they have changed, or have they? Does Doctor Dear (male or female) believe as Ring Lardner, Jr.'s character who said, "Women should be kept illiterate and clean, like canaries." Do they believe as Guy, who turns to his wife Olivia in *Fortunes of War* seen last year on public television and says, "You have a job. I have WORK."

That's what the administrators and doctors and big business used to think about nurses. And ten years from now I am going to stand in front of some audience somewhere and say, "That's what they used to think about medical transcriptionists." As some wag said, "Doctors will get off their pedestals when patients get off their knees." That also works when medical transcription businesses do the same.

Doctor, doctor, doctor—Well, I never count my doctors before they are hatched, but today is different. I begin reaching for my drug of choice, Pepto-Bismol, before broaching this subject. Will doctors change? Can they change? Will many of them feel forever that Medical Records is some Black Hole of Calcutta, some Bermuda Triangle of disaster where their perfectly good dictated reports are lost forever amid moans and sighs? Will the young fresh ones, male and female, ever stop chewing gum and eating lunch and learn to say thank you, or is my cry going to go unheeded for another dusty canyon of years?

Can we blame the doctor for feeling cheated by tradesmen who pad the bill because they figure the rich doctor can afford it, so when the doctor talks with the medical transcription service, that attitude carries over?

Can doctors deal with obscene insurance rates in the morning and then with a reasonable transcription rate in the afternoon? Or will the doctor give me that wry lemony smile while hissing, "Well, Mrs. Marshall, if you had the superjet pow-pow laser printer, my work could be done six times as fast and you could fax the H&Ps or send by modem," and I hiss back, "But doctor, dear doctor, if we did that you would be paying us $4.00 a line for all this glorious technology."

How would we feel if the insurance industry set our rates, then gave us 80 percent of that payment? Ah, but I digress into my usual full-blown hyperbole.

Working in a hospital and nursing, of course, were considered practically religious vocations in the early days, and transcription had its saints and martyrs. Women who threw themselves on tapes like a soldier throwing himself on a live grenade to save his comrades.

Then something changed, even before Medicare in 1965.

The bloom was off the rose.

The frost was off the pumpkin.

The glamour was off the puss.

The work force began to change.

Technology began to change and for hospitals it was time to wake up and smell the Betadine. Like the British in India who taught the Indians, in the 19th century, their own history and their own culture, the British who tried to build roads and restore monuments and drag the sleepy continent into the 20th century, American business came to the hospital. It was the businessmen who noted the unit of measurement as a way to revolutionize medical transcription and to make it more efficient and cost-effective by moving it off-site or putting production workers on-site.

NOT FOR PROFIT!

I feel more pain when I hear this than a vampire does upon having a stake driven through his heart. Also, because I never believed hospitals were not for profit—to me it was often an excuse for slipshod business practices.

When business moved into medical transcription, I was ready. The seduction really began in Medical Records with one doctor and one little bitty tape. I can remember him holding the tape, standing behind me. "Do this for me tonight," he said, "and I will make it worth your while." The scent of money rose from his expensive clothes and I was hooked. Note how women thought and STILL think. Not "How can I get a raise?" (locked into the hospital grading system) but "How many more hours can I work?"

And what a schizophrenic business! Business people in competition with non-business people. Is there any other business that operates like ours on TWO levels? I, a service owner, am in competition with three someones who undercharge, underbid, and underperform in quality and turnaround. The hospital says, "Why not deliver three times a day? *They* do." "Why not spell out all abbreviations, even the word 'doctor'? *They* do." "Why not wait 120 days to get paid? *They* do."

How have MTs changed and how are we as employers to cope?

1. They are angrier—a feeling of powerlessness, helplessness—and many off-site transcriptionists never saw the whole picture or had any input into, say, the purchase of new equipment or change of forms they themselves use daily.

2. They are more demanding in terms of money but even more so in terms of flextime, formatting, keeping logs, and so on.

3. Many MTs for the FIRST TIME are being monitored by computer for keystroke, line, page, whatever, and they really resent it. And many for the first time are pitted against what the off-site transcription service is doing. The hospital workers learn quickly to hate the off-site service people. Here is the golden opportunity for the service owner to find the MT who is a great production worker or one who would be agreeable to base pay and incentive. The business can operate on two concurrent pay methods or switch between the two. The hospital bureaucracy makes that less likely.

4. The American Association for Medical Transcription has changed thousands of MTs. Imagine putting five hundred women in a hotel for four days at a national meeting in

a vocal, articulate, consciousness-raising environment, and letting them talk and share information until they drop. AAMT gave what was once only a job a position of esteem and visibility. The good employers will love AAMT and the not-so-good will want their staffs isolated and uninformed.

5. Technology has created a new pool of workers who are computer literate and keyboard masters. (That would make a good company name, Keyboard Masters.) This current situation coincides with the new tools of teaching and software and books from Health Professions Institute, Prima Vera Publications, AAMT, W.B. Saunders, and many, many others.

It is hoped that with these new tools we can put an end to the "rabbit ventricular response" and the "chronic Venice (or Venus) insufficiency." Unless the MT really reads and loves words, no computer will help, I suppose.

So, what, to paraphrase Freud, do medical transcriptionists want, anyway? They want acceptance. They want reward, status, and recognition. They want money, yes, but they really want more time off. They want more flexible schedules. They want better benefits. They want better working conditions and better equipment. They want better resources, books, and in-service education, and they will often gravitate to work for a business which provides some hope of advancement. They want clear samples and formats. They want current doctor lists. They want as little clerical work as possible if they are production people. They want one boss, not several. And they want an end to the Mommy Manager.

I wish us all an end to the Mommy Manager. I got a note last year attached to some work. It said, "Judith, this is a no-no." I felt tiny and defenseless. I was a child again. I had pee-peed in my po-po and gotten caught.

The Mommy Manager tends to make sprawling negative statements to your company. The phone call that says,

"That last batch had several errors." Oh, please, we have it all on disk—what errors, where? Work with us to correct any errors. We have spent years whipping our staffs into shape and we do good work. Criticism must be *specific*.

I hope this conference will help us to become more effective managers ourselves while dealing with the Mommy Managers. For example, when we have a new client, a lucrative, difficult, wacky format, a dictating cast of thousands, and we perform brilliantly, the RRA calls and says, "Well, you didn't leave enough space for the signature and the doctors are complaining." Does it take an MBA from Harvard to know that if you told that to your staff, they would probably walk out?

Now, I asked myself, why did we all come here to San Francisco? Women call me and say, "I just love this business. How DID you do it?" In the past I had told them ALL, and only after many years and much wasted time did I begin to say, "Look, get a lawyer, get a good accountant, get an ad agency and a pile of capital and go, baby!"

So why SHOULD big business talk to little business or medium business talk to solo self-employeds? I think because a meeting like this enhances all of our images in the public eye as well as intra-industry. Because the exchange of information is worth the trip. Because we are a diverse group of employables and resources for learning. And because AMRA and AAMT are not enough.

Want a piece of candy, little girl? You bet I do. And the sweetshop is HERE.

Summer 1990

Is Medical Transcription a Laughing Matter?

Straight talk
to Medical Record Directors

Alvin Toffler's book *Third Wave* published in 1980 predicted a shift from an industrial society to a technologic information-oriented society, millions of Americans telecommuting and making the home the dominant site of all human activity, work and play. I would be interested in the results of the 1990 census (if they ever pick up all the forms), but there seem to be about 26 million Americans working at home, with 6 million of them telecommuting full-time.

Many of you know that the AFL-CIO and other labor unions are vehemently opposed to telecommuting as a loss to the member base, I believe, and the inability to control the labor force; independent contractors without any benefits, with their own means of production, paid on piecework rates—the so-called Electronic Cottage, or the Electronic Sweatshop.

That's a pretty bleak summary. On the other hand, a highly-motivated medical transcriptionist with state-of-the-art technology, connected to the hospital by the invisible golden threads of modern communication, able to be monitored for quality control, with printing done in the hospital—all can combine to increase your employee stability and decrease turnaround time as well as chip away at the increasing benefit costs. This is still a women-dominated business. I recognize there are men working along with us— may their numbers increase and thus wages will rise for all of us. This women-dominated field can be a great boon to the hospital employer. A worker in the last trimester of pregnancy or convalescing from a hysterectomy—not quite ready to schlepp to the workplace but happy to telecommute—here is a resource we have just begun to tap.

You are no longer limited to advertising in the local paper or the *Boston Globe*. AMRA and AAMT publications, *For the Record*, *Perspectives*, and *Transcription Today* offer national ads.

Base pay plus incentive becomes more of a reality, and with technology counting for you (nothing new here; we had cyclometers twenty years ago), how grand it is. I believe medical transcription will be measured increasingly by character counts, automatically done by computer software.

I have often been asked whether I find this sort of measuring and piecework demeaning and repugnant. Not at all. I am a production worker by nature. Another way to put it might be that I am an obsessive-compulsive maniac and can't resist transcription, which is my chance to create order around me and build defenses in my environment against an insane world.

If you do add to your staff and choose telecommuters, the professionals tell us to choose those who have already worked on site, people who are highly motivated production workers and get along well with others. I believe they should be *employees*—with benefits as well as the chance to advance. I have always believed in staff meetings, creating them in the face of very angry resistance in one hospital in Boston where the staff had to come in a half hour earlier once every two weeks. Even with three shifts, this can be done at least monthly. This promotes the team and the concepts of shared responsibilities and heightened commitment.

Personally, I believe the best transcription by the best people with the best effect for patient care is done by your staff in your hospital. That is less heresy than you may think for someone of my ilk. Realistically, how can a hospital provide coverage for radiology on a Sunday? Bring the transcriptionist in to cover or have the digital dictation system accessed by several transcriptionists taking turns on a Sunday? Whoever takes a Sunday gets some time off equal to the transcription time—no high cost of double time. But we'd better hurry. Voice-activated dictation will take this over very soon in the radiology department.

So, are the same tired menopausal women being recycled from place to place? Not necessarily.

Medical records directors will be making decisions about their services off-site and about digital dictation costs—who is paying for the tie-lines, the telephone charges, the unit charges for the black box units, perhaps who pays for extra disks. Your bills may reflect higher costs for laser printers purchased by the service. Are these offset by the hospital's savings on expensive printed forms? Technology is fabulous but it is expensive and the set-up charges can be astronomical.

There are many problems with digital dictation. If I can dial in for the oldest dictation and there are 15 ports and other workers dialing in, we can keep it current and modem back the work. But if the hospital is using digital dictation and getting backed up in transcription and has to download or re-record in real time, all of us are going backwards.

What a fresh breeze of freedom, too, in telecommuting when the telephone charges are low from 11 p.m. to 7 a.m. and the worker who was terrified to come into the inner city for that shift, or is snowed in, or does not drive (yes, there are still some) is now happy, awake, and working for YOU all night long.

I always say the heart of the hospital is the medical records department but don't tell that to the personnel

department—excuse me, the department of human resources. If they control the advertising, they control the
wording of the copy and they control the people whom you
will see. This is a mixed blessing.

How are transcriptionists classified in your institution? If
they are still clerk-typists, medical secretaries, or if the job
description includes telephone answering and photocopying, recruiting can be difficult. Every time I see a skilled production worker doing clerical functions, that is to me a dollar
doing a nickel's work. It is tough to buck administration and
to rewrite job descriptions, but I think it is the first step to a
truly fine transcription section.

And please, please, please, let's kill the typing test. Great
transcriptionists are often unable to copy-type one sentence
correctly. Typesetters who can copy Hungarian with complete diacritical marks have trouble acclimating to the transcription mode. To test a transcriptionist, have a tape
(perhaps 15 minutes' worth of dictation) transcribed.

Training is easier than it used to be. If you have the
costs figured, if you have the environment, the space, and
the ability to absorb or overcome all the extra noise and
interruption—now is better than ever to train your own.
Why? Because we have tools we never had. The American
Association for Medical Transcription and Health Professions
Institute have created systems of real dictation on tape
accompanied by transcript keys which take the novice from
the simple to the complex.

Let's also kill the terminology courses that go on for two
years, bringing me candidates who know that "itis" means
inflammation but can't sit down and transcribe it. Let's learn
by doing. Publishers have produced word books that are
unparalleled in their accuracy and ease of use.

When I see a department with a shredded and torn old
Stedman's and a 1987 *PDR*, I can imagine the quality of the

transcription. I tell people if I were on a desert island with my work, I would take my *American Drug Index* by Billups and my Saunders' and Health Professions Institute's word books and software. *Stedman's* is now in software, of course. Macros are fraught with dangers but when used wisely can aid production and quality.

A major problem in training I have seen in departments and services is when lead transcriptionists or senior staff are the "helpers" or "trainers" and are not paid for this extra duty, nor is it part of their job description. At first these folks may feel flattered but often they end up being increasingly hostile, bothered, and resentful. Another problem is saving easy transcription for the beginners while the old battle-axes, your veterans of many wars, are still struggling with Dr. Bunofuna, the ophthalmologist from Pakistan, or Dr. Tex from the West Pecos.

While your transcription service is well paid to do what you send them, they also know when you are sending out the worst; these days, services are charging more for that. When I receive 3000 minutes of dictation, 70% of which is ancient dictation of Dr. Wojciehowicz, I know they saved it for me. Even if my relatives sound just like him, this is a pain in the gluteus maximus and my billing is renegotiated to reflect this.

I think there is a less adversarial feeling between the AMRA people and the transcription service people in the last few years, but we have a way to go. All of us have been forced to accept rapid technological change and a younger workforce less committed today to ideals than we are.

I myself deal with many service owners and am embarrassed for them. A woman who runs a business grossing $200,000+ answers the phone with the baby in her arms, and I have to say hello to the baby so she will be quiet and then I can deal with the mother. Well, what sort of professional image is that?

Women who show up at the Palmer House in Chicago in blue jeans, snapping their fingers at the waiter and calling him "garcon." Women who call their staffs "my girls" (one of my pet peeves) give me visions of fields of pickaninnies in bandannas laboring under the hot sun, or a roomful of children in nappies. To me, professionalism BEGINS with nomenclature.

Services have to become more lean and mean as they invest more capital in technology. They are not going to burst and collate and archive and keep logs and look up referring physician names or addresses of hospitals out of state—or they will, but they will charge heavily for it.

Three kinds of services seem to exist: (1) We will do anything, anything, for a price. (2) We will not do just anything, but we will negotiate almost everything. (3) If it is WRONG, we will not do it, period; for example, spell out the word DOCTOR and the word MILLIGRAMS in every sentence in every report in every instance.

Conversely, we will not shorten and abbreviate all the words to reduce the stroke count, as in "pt. adm. to hos." You think I make up these things? I have both real cases in my files. Does the same Joint Commission that I know peek at these records at all?

I will fight indenting and underlining and multiple forms in various colors, forms with lines on them (type on the line, they say, as if we are using typewriters these days). I will ask questions, and sometimes that is hard for a director to accept. And the answer "We have always done it this way" is difficult for me to accept when I know how much it is costing, or that it is just a whim of someone probably retired now, or just plain bad form.

Medical record directors have a great deal of power and prestige and I am often in awe of them. I wish they would all realize that power and use it. Directors have the power to deal with the physicians—the fast talkers who are impossible to transcribe, the slobs, the abusers of stat lines, the residents dictating 10-page summaries, the deliberate coding of 999 by doctors who just want to get into the system. Many physicians can and will change when they are properly approached and have costs explained to them. Perhaps they are not so unwilling to cooperate, just ignorant of the system.

Before the days of telecommuting, when couriers were used to deliver work to the hospital, one of our unhappiest moments was finding the bag of work from the day before, just lying there, unprocessed. I would say, "Look, if you can't get to it, at least hide it from us."

Lastly, if you have a contract or a verbal agreement, your service should not be having problems with Accounts Payable. If there are problems, a supportive manager helps. I hate to call Accounts Payable, but recently I did to ask about a $1400 check. The clerk said to me, "What kind of business are you running that a $1400 check matters so much you have to call us long distance about it?" Excuse me? I called the director of medical records. She said she felt the clerk was not out of line. We don't do business with that hospital anymore.

At a recent medical transcription industry conference, it was interesting to see how many service owners now would hold a client's tapes hostage or the work hostage, if their bills were not paid by the client. They said they would hold things without a qualm, after a certain point, expressly stating that in the contract.

So who has the last laugh? You and your on-site healthcare team of transcriptionists or your home-sweet-office telecommuting staff? Or those of you with off-premises total contract service? I hope all of us do.

October 1990

Flow Gently, Sweet Barium

I should have known better. I worked for a screwball in the first radiology account a few years ago. He was wiry and good-looking and owned his own x-ray company. We danced around the topics of price and turnaround time and made little jokes about opening a bar we would call "Luschka's Joint" next door to the ophthalmology practice, "The Eyes Have It." I remember thinking, "Get a grip, Marshall. You get involved with this man and you will absorb enough radiation to light up Chicago." There never was an affair, but there was an account. He turned out to be a scatter-brained, ferret-faced deadbeat whom I sued in Small Claims Court (and won).

When the second radiology account came my way and the director outlined the specs, I was very happy. It was a simple deal. The hospital had installed a new digital dictation system but the radiologists refused to use it. In fact, they never even changed their own tapes in their hand-held recorders. A courier would bring tapes and requisitions to me (between 4:30 p.m. and as late as 10:45 p.m., as it evolved). I would transcribe at night but could not transmit via modem until 7:30 a.m. when their day shift came on.

At first that seemed reasonable. Months later, it became a nightmare. I was convinced they would honor the contract and I would be able to access their printer directly, without the staff person there having to ring my computer first. That never happened.

Months earlier when I went there for a mammogram, a warning bell rang which I ignored. I asked for a copy of my report and was told by the clerk that this was "forbidden." I called Medical Records and they told me to sign the release, pay the ten dollars, and I could have a copy for myself. The R.T. said if I were using deodorant or talcum powder that day, I would be given soap and towel and sent to bathe.

I asked the same clerk, a veritable fount of information, why I was not told in advance about abstaining from talcum and deodorant for a mammogram. Surely this was a common requirement and easy enough to tell a patient when the appointment was booked. Wide-eyed, the clerk exclaimed, "Wow, you sure are teaching me a lot today and I have been here for two years!" Now that I was damp and late for my next appointment, I retorted, "I should not be teaching you anything. I am just a patient. You people ought to learn this from your supervisors."

So I had known there were sloppy clerical practices and ill-trained personnel behind the desk. I took the account anyway.

The dictators were two Grand Masters of Dark Shadows. One was monotonous, the other sprightly. One had never learned his Latin endings so every dictation was sprinkled with ACETABULEE and DIVERTICULEE. The other made puns of patient names, probably to avoid going insane with boredom. Once in a while someone would hit a moose on the highway or be kicked by a cow or stick his hand in a chainsaw or ski into a tree, but most reports were fairly routine.

A patient named Maud had a chest x-ray, and this fellow sang the theme song from the TV show, "And here comes Maud—with her chest." Or the indication on a hip x-ray, "Fell down. Go boom." Neither ever said thank you. When I asked to meet the physicians, I was brushed off. "We never bother our doctors."

Heckel and Jeckel (the two clerks) had never worked in a hospital or a business setting. As often happens in bureaucracies, the lower rungs see it's their god-given right to crush the bottom rung (in this case, the off-site transcription service). The battles were about handwriting on the requisitions. Some sheets had as many as four people writing on them. The worst penmanship belonged to the doctors (no surprise there), and the worst of the doctors was the one who admitted the most patients. This was the same guy who would order a lot of routine chest x-rays on his female patients over 40 and enter the clinical diagnosis as "Depression. Neurosis." Once in a while he would add ''Cough and fever."

I told the clerks if the data was illegible, it would not appear on the report. The clerks said everything was plain enough and why not call and ask them if I had a question. Why must addresses and phone numbers and other decorative garnish appear on every report? The man with the terrible handwriting wanted it that way. I felt myself regressing into a sandbox state of mind, and all of us were two years old and fighting with plastic pails and shovels.

The months dragged on. To amuse myself, I named my directory Dem Bones. Each day's file became T-Bone or Lamb Chop, Hambone or Wishbone. After I ran out of bones, I went on to flowers and proclaimed the sweetpea the national flower of urologists.

After six months the director called to berate me about all the missing data and errors her "girls" found every day. She complained that the LMPs (last menstrual periods) were missing "on most of these." She lectured to me about risk management, as if there are a thousand court cases a year based on radiation-deformed fetuses. I told her I had photocopied all the requisitions; which LMPs were missing? That ended that. What were the errors? Everything is on the disk, I told her, and we are happy to redo or rerun reports at no charge, but the lady was not happy about anything. The contract expired and the hospital wanted to renew. My instincts told me to decline.

Lack of communication can kill an account. I should have been much more assertive in meeting with the clerical staff at the first whiff of flatulence. I should have insisted upon meeting the physicians.

There is a larger issue here. Perhaps that is why I have a sense of loss as acute as over the man who got away in 1967. This was an opportunity for the hospital to use its marvelous and expensive technology. Radiology reports could be dictated on a digital system, transcribed almost immediately seven days a week, and returned by modem to their printer. What formerly took their employee eight hours took me initially five hours, then with the use of a macro system, two hours per day.

Why were so many requisitions 48 to 72 hours old before I even got them? Why not dictate inpatient reports first? Why was management so sensitive to the perceived needs of doctors and why was management afraid to place emphasis on patient care by faster turnaround of reports? If the report was not on the chart or available to the internist, the transcription service was to blame, of course.

Heckel and Jeckel only mirrored the attitudes of management and were poorly trained as well. They have gone back to whatever it is they do. The hospital paid for state-of-the-art equipment and has people who will not or cannot use it effectively.

I have a microwave I don't know how to use and I never learned to program the VCR, but who cares what I do in my house? Healthcare consumers, however, pay more because of situations like this. Well, flow gently, sweet barium, but now without me.

May 1991

Call Me Madam

Those twenty dwarfs turning handstands on the carpet of my mind must be medical transcriptionists. With the temperature at minus 29 degrees I am getting a little bugsy myself and more than hyperalert at the computer.

Is the content of the medical dictation changing for the worse or am I just suffering contact dermatitis from Tide in those new little boxes?

There is an increase in the use of first names, not just in psychiatric summaries but in all specialties. A 71-year-old female enters the hospital for *rule out myocardial infarction* and the doctor tells us "Fiona" did this and that. If Fiona is from a nursing home, the chances increase dramatically that her surname will be amputated. The older a male patient becomes, the more likely is he to be called by his first name.

If a patient is admitted for drug or alcohol detoxification or any AIDS-related reason, the use of first names increases. I don't think it is a matter of confidentiality. I think it is a matter of doctors doing (pardon me, George) "the power thing."

For the past thirty years, I have been listening to the Ob-Gyn doctors and one has to give them an A in consistency. They are still patronizing as heck, though they are much more democratic now and have progressed beyond the "little mothers." More women are practicing in obstetrics and gynecology and, unfortunately, have developed a style of "manly" dictation, i.e., using the patient's first name. All those nurse-midwives fought so hard in so many places for the right to be part of the hospital medical team. Then they dictate using the woman's first name, and oy, we are up to our ankles in girl stuff.

Am I the only sentinel? Are there other "first name police" out there? Weren't we trained never to transcribe the patient's name in the body of a report? Not for anyone, not even for babies and children. Is this a question of form, content, ethics, manners, or, heaven help us, total quality? Does AAMT or AHIMA think about these things?

In the McDonaldization of American medical language as practiced in dictating summaries, there seems to be less consideration, kindness, and, yes, morality when dealing with human suffering. What, in person, can be a ploy to ameliorate the dehumanizing technological aspect of medical care becomes, on paper, plain crass.

In routine long-term transcription for a sixtyish gentleman internist, I dutifully type his "chronic anxiety-depression syndrome" diagnosis for all his female patients over forty. Since the women never see the reports, I suppose they never know. The transcription supervisor told me he appeared on Valentine's Day morning and asked her why she wasn't wearing red. "I like to see all of my girls in red today."

After the Clarence Thomas/Anita Hill brouhaha, why should I get my pantyhose in a twist over the use of first names in medical reports?

Because what I am talking about is basic human dignity. Because when formal hospital documents become chatty and palsy-walsy and careless and sloppy, it worries me. And when a patient is bare-bottomed, poked, prodded, sedated, and confused, that is especially when he needs to be a *Mister*, not just *Joe*. A woman in diapers or bleeding through her clothes or being examined status post mastectomy needs to be a *Missus*, not just *Kathy*.

Last week I visited a friend who had cardiac surgery in a major Boston teaching hospital. He handed me his discharge summary. It was printed all in caps, with abbreviations from the diagnoses to the last sentence. "THE PT. WAS AD. TO THE HOS." The lengthy discharge diagnoses were all abbreviated. Hello, Joint Commission?

I called a woman in the biz who knows the area. She said the hospital was encouraging the residents to sit at the screen and peck out their summaries and paying them a couple of bucks to do it. "All they want is the record, Judith," she said. "Never mind anything else."

Next time you visit your doctor, see how the secretary addresses you. If it is by your first name, correct her. Then correct the doctor. It is a short hip-hop from name to attitude.

November 1991

"And the Corral Sang On"— Raising Cultural Literacy in the Profession

Adapted from a speech presented to teachers of medical transcription at a seminar in Chicago on April 30, 1992, sponsored by Health Professions Institute.

How to raise cultural literacy? As a teacher, you make decisions about textbooks, word books, and methodology that will help translate cultural literacy to the work world and enhance the linguistic and scientific aspects of teaching medical transcription.

In the '80s, Letterperfect Medical Transcription was a doctor-based service near Boston, with more than 250 accounts. A doctor in a solo practice often seeks out a transcription service for excellence. He tends to be highly critical of what he is signing and he reads before he signs.

We worked for a brilliant physician, a client with many interests, including the Boston Symphony. He wrote a letter to Seiji Ozawa and praised him for the holiday program including "handles mesiuh, especially the corral." The transcriptionist never asked, the proofreader sailed right over it, and the client was apoplectic with rage at our "letting him down." The MT spelled phonetically, a situation which we label the conceit of ignorance. I thought the proofreader knew better as she was a voracious reader and a summa

61

cum laude college graduate. She confessed she had scanned a few reports since they were always the same. She missed the business letter.

My office was technologically complete. The staff was highly motivated. The lighting, ergonomic necessities, chairs, headphones, reference books, spellcheckers, PRD+— all were at the ready. Then some doctor goes to a concert, gets a bug up his stethoscope to praise the orchestra, and the end result is what I call "the puu-puu platter of errors." This corral was definitely not O.K.

My neighbor, a regular Ms. Malaprop, was discussing the summer tourists, or "flatlanders" who invade Vermont. Some of the hippie element camp near graveyards where there are no facilities. My neighbor cried out, "Oh, Judith, I just hate it when these gippies [her cross between a gypsy and a hippie] come and defamate in our beautiful cemeteries."

Our society's education or lack thereof affects all of us at all levels, and it is from this societal pool our students come. General knowledge is lacking in all sectors of our economy and daily life.

Do you watch television? Admit it. Not public television. Commercial television. Have you wondered why *Wayne's World* and *Home Alone* grossed more than predicted? Was it appeal to the lowest common denominator of national intelligence or because only young people were buying tickets? Two major megacorporations are battling to sell Pepsi Cola and Coca-Cola and the slogans their millions bought from the ad agencies were UH-HUH and GOTTA HAVE IT.

If EuroDisney is a "cultural Chernobyl," whose culture are the French intellectuals disparaging, mes infants? Disney stock is now at $152 a share and rising.

In our classrooms and in daily life, we want the person who reads. I ask students to list what newspapers and magazines they read regularly and what books they read lately. I want to know if they like film and go to the movies or rent videos. I ask them which movies they have seen lately or what they like. Do they watch *Jeopardy*?

Medical transcriptionists traditionally did not require higher education. We are now in the midst of an era which demands it. Just as an ART and RRA must grapple with more than the technical aspects of data, educators and business owners must look to educated people, not just keyboard wizards. Educated people cost money. They ask questions. They exude professionalism. They love learning. They want to do a good job. We are moving away from the days when someone could "pick up" the medical lingo by sitting next to someone and many hospitals called it their "training program."

AHIMA and AAMT recognize that continuing education makes the professional. Otherwise we are all chipmunks on an exercise wheel, with great speed, enviable industriousness, but essentially going nowhere in a one-track world.

Susan Turley wrote two articles which are germane to this discussion: "Improving Our Vocabulary: English Words" published in the *Journal of AAMT*, Fall 1985, in which she stressed the use of the dictionary in teaching and gave a sample test of English vocabulary; and "Medical Literacy," in *Perspectives*, Winter 1991-92, exploring that theme further and encouraging teachers to create an atmosphere where questions on all levels are valid. There is no such thing as a stupid question, in other words.

I thought I had created that atmosphere in my business. But the transcriptionist did not ask about the chorale which sang Handel's *Messiah*. Did I fail her or did my system fail her? Now that I have more experience, I think the way she was paid (on production), the big buck for the short haul, impeded her from stopping and getting those fingers off the keyboard and into a dictionary.

In teaching or in the workplace, one can plead and cajole and then as a final resort, pull out the club of authority and beat people to a pulp. It doesn't work. If formal authority comes from above and informal authority or earned authority comes from below, our success at any level is dependent upon the success of our subordinates. We are all responsible for that success in our subordinates. The club is really not an option.

I would like a classroom or office atmosphere to be a place where people learn to think. And if they THINK they do not KNOW, then they will leave a BLANK and ASK. Then we are successful.

Some suggestions for increasing cultural literacy are:

1. **Encourage reading of anything and everything**, from the tabloids to the *Wall Street Journal*, magazines, medical journals, *Journal of AAMT*, *Journal of AHIMA*, *Perspectives*. Encourage discussion of material taken from current women's magazines and health columns of weeklies and newspapers. Use bulletin boards.

2. **Never laugh at any question**. As Vera Pyle wrote, ''A blank is an honorable thing. It means you don't know.''

3. **If you are including grammar, try to use real examples from medical reports**. I attended an AAMT symposium where the lecturer on grammar was a fabulous and vivacious teacher. But all the examples were of nonmedical sentences and rendered the topic dull. The next day I was transcribing and heard, "He sees an outpatient therapist who speaks Chinese every two weeks." And it clicked! How effective all the same material would have been with medical examples.

4. **Quality assurance.** Quality checks in a systematic routine fashion will pinpoint errors and categorize them into English errors, medical terminology errors, surgical terminology errors, etc. Quality checks done against the tape are preferred to proofing alone. This, of course, depends upon the system one is using to teach.

5. **Red flags and red herrings**.

a. **Doctors who are dictating out of their specialty**. The patient was admitted to Gynecology and has surgery. But the patient also has a podiatric problem with recurrent infection. The dictating doctor will know his own specialty but may be lost outside of it and to be helpful will try to spell, usually incorrectly.

b. **ESL** (English as a second language) **physicians**. And not for the reasons you think. It may not be their accent at all that is the problem. Some of them are guessing. And they are stringing together sounds and fudging. How do I know? I have done the same thing. I had to learn other languages. In Polish, I would say "mianowicie," which means "namely," and lengthened my sentence. I was fudging. ESL physicians sometimes try to be cool and run things together. In surgical dictation, they might say "Following this" four hundred times. They love abbreviations without knowing what they mean. When they say "hint" for HEENT or even H-E-E-N-T, then say "head, eyes, ears, nose, and throat," I know I have them by the tail.

c. **Business letters**. "And the corral sang on." Need I say more?

d. **Psychiatry/substance abuse**. "The patient inhaled kiln coating and saw angels dancing on the head of a pin." The long and reflective nature of many psychiatric reports provides a rich vocabulary challenge to the most jaded of transcriptionists. The proportion of slang is increased in these reports, so the possibility of error increases as well. The street names for drugs are varied and challenging. Even the social history can be challenging. Women are widows, men are widowers. *Fiance*, male, has one *e*; *fiancee*, female, has two.

e. It is not enough to provide the student a copy of Billups' *American Drug Index*; **the student must learn how to** *use* **references**. In the back of the book there is an excellent section on unique packaging trademarks such as Dosepak. Also, I have met many people who don't know that the drugs marked with a black dot throughout the *Drug Index* are generic drugs. Teachers must be familiar with their resources.

Education is, after all, sometimes just connecting the dots of varied experiences, relating facts we already know. I spoke at a symposium in which a doctor lectured about herpes, to which I never had paid much attention. He looked just like Al Pacino and came from Brooklyn. It was a good lecture with good slides. I finally learned about the terrible disease and its effects. And I thought about the old days when we worried about halitosis and clean sheets as we bed-hopped. Now that people are walking around with lethal weapons in their underpants, it is very sobering. Which led me to think about Scott Turow's novel, *The Burden of Proof.* So I asked the audience who had read it. One woman had and she knew that the motive for the suicide involved an extramarital affair, the contraction of herpes, and the pain and suffering afterward. This connection of bits of facts now became a solid learning experience.

We all want the same thing. The pursuit of excellence—you betcha. The achievement of excellence—you betcha. When the *New England Journal of Medicine*, the *New York Times*, the *Wall Street Journal*, the *Washington Post*, NBC, ABC, CBS, CNN, and Masterpiece Theater don't care anymore, we will care.

When Vice President Dan Quayle says they speak Latin in Latin America and everyone believes him and doesn't laugh, I will know he is wrong and so will you. I'm glad we are colleagues. We care about what is correct and accurate. We don't want anyone to defamate in the medical record.

May 1992

Doctors 10
Handmaidens . 0

For some time I have been fascinated with how health information managers (HIMs) cope with the angst of chart completion. Earlier this year *Advance*, a biweekly for HIMs and others in allied healthcare fields, published a story about one hospital department's methodology. They installed a putting green for the physicians as an incentive to record completion. Another hospital had a luau!

Coffee and cake I had heard of, but this was beyond my wildest dreams. What happened to the medical staff doing their job like everyone else? What were these sophomoric good ole boys and gals doing? And why were HIMs allowing it? This daffy approach does not help the doctor image, either. "Have some food, my children," the Mommy Manager says, "and this unpalatable task will go down easier."

Daniel Buchak, ART, of Elmhurst, New York, wrote to *Advance* with the revolutionary idea of solving the problem through "effective use of medical stiff by-laws and communication among medical records staff, physicians, and administrators." "Physicians should complete records out of a sense of responsibility to the patients and their peers." And he got smacked right on his naughty little hands by the editor of *Advance* who chided him, saying the luau was ONLY a one-time event and that life being what it is, physicians do not always do the right thing, telling Buchak to lighten up and foster a spirit of cooperation and communication "with a little humor."

Now I was really interested. I called Buchak, who said he had had a very positive feedback from other HIMs about his stance and stated he was "an optimist but not panglossian." Buchak is Director of Clinical Information Management at his facility. He went on to cite what he called "the ridiculous pandering to physicians," and I knew I was in love.

Buchak's focus was on the redundancy and intricacy of forms which waste doctors' time and increase their frustration. "Don't give them donuts or pizza," he said. "Give them less to write." About one issue, Buchak waffled and was reluctant to speak. I asked him if this were a case of the nearly all-female medical records staff fluttering over the nearly all-male medical staff. It reminded me of "File Under G for Gravy," which I wrote in July 1989 about "the idea of the medical transcriptionist as the handmaiden of medical records." "She kissed so many backsides, she suffered from bunburn."

William F. Doran, RRA, Director of Information Services at Boston City Hospital, took the issue and throttled it blue. Recognizing the female-dominated RRAs and ARTs, Doran wrote to *Advance* that parties and the like "undeniably prolong and continue to foster the belief that the HIM field is a handmaiden to the currently male-dominated field of medicine." Here is obviously a person averse to hiney-kissing.

The debate continues. Wilma Holland of Transcription Services in Annadale, Virginia, wrote, "What happened to the old work ethic—shape up or ship out?" Debra Kister, RRA, of Fox Chase Cancer Center in Philadelphia, suggested having adequate work space for physicians to complete records, with personnel and systems resources readily available. Cynthia Chicker, RRA, The Richland Hospital in Richland

Center, Wisconsin, does use "contests, an occasional conti-
nental breakfast," and calls this "positive reinforcement."
"The bottom line seems to be what matters, not how you
get there." I beg to differ. It matters very much how one gets
there.

Software may be an answer. The May 1992 *Journal of
AHIMA* published an ad for National Healthcare Review with
a cartoon of a woman running after a doctor and the caption says, "If you're tired of chasing doctors, we've got a
system for you."

The lively exchange in *Advance* shows that societal as
well as hospital attitudes accept the fallacy that doctors
wear royal purple and the rest of the peasants, especially
female peasants, serve the doctors. I believe that, when presented with rational business logic and systems, physicians
can and will cooperate with even the most pedestrian
aspects of their work. And when that fails, other systems,
such as admitting privileges or paycheck withholding, if
enforced equitably, must be employed.

Attitudes of power and privilege permeate the entire
bureaucracy of medical records. When dictating systems
were introduced, doctors soon learned that if they punched
all nines instead of the patient number, they could enter the
system without furrowing their brows. Why give patient
demographic information if the trolls under the bridge in
Medical Records will fill it in? HIMs often use the stock
phrase, "We don't bother the doctors." Hospitals spend an
inordinate amount of money on clerical efforts to rectify
what could have been dictated correctly in the first place. Of
course, new software is helping change this.

When I was naive enough to believe that hospitals existed
for the welfare of patients, great dinosaurs roamed the earth.
Hospitals were created to benefit the doctors. Will doctors
continue to operate above the law, so to speak? As long as

they are rewarded for not complying in the first place, I think so. Strong managers are required to correct centuries of sexism and kowtowing to false idols.

There is often a direct ratio between the number of patients a physician admits and the degree of laxity in medical records completion. "My hands are tied," says Administration. "Let's keep the doctor happy."

My editor is screaming for this article but I told her I want a cookie first, many, many cookies. My clients are screaming for turnaround and I told them to send flowers or wait. I want rewards before I do my job. Ray Pinder, RRA, Hospital of Philadelphia, College of Osteopathy, would understand. He announced a glittery incentive for chart completion. Pinder is having a weekly drawing for dinner tickets to the hospital dinner dance, including limousine service.

May 1992

Bye Bye, Ball

Late September in the Northeast Kingdom of Vermont has a luscious beauty that makes the heart ache. The light is tilted slightly, the air is azure and thick with frenzied green things growing and ending in sweet harvest. There is a haze over the mountains and the tips of the maples are brilliantly reddened, like elegant old ladies with crimson nails, determined to be beautiful until the end.

There is a September of the soul as well. Growing older means letting go of some dreams and rituals. It means we will never read all the books we had planned, embroider all the pillow cases in the drawer, or make all the recipes in the file.

I suppose I never will learn to water ski or play the cello or speak French fluently. And now I have to face the fact that I will never learn to can. Ball Corporation announced in August it is getting out of the home canning business after 112 years.

Folkways change and are lost almost as imperceptibly as the summer yields to autumn. I hang out the wash which evokes some atavistic female satisfaction, as I imagine generations of women in hundreds of cultures, clucking approval as they pin the laundry to billow in the wind. My city friends laugh at me but I don't care.

Mundane shopping becomes a primal rush to forage, gather and return to the cave, clutching my treasures. Ironing linen and polishing silver are tranquil tasks and pleasing to me. In a world where everything is becoming sanitized, packed, pre-measured, plastic-wrapped, and bar-coded, I remember a different and slower time.

Fifty years ago, in an immaculate basement in a Cleveland neighborhood called Warszawa, I sat quietly with my girlhood chum and watched her mother and aunt canning. There were heaps of produce laying on newspapers and water boiling on an ancient black stove. The sisters spoke in rapid Polish and were dressed for battle in housedresses and crisp, full aprons.

Bushel baskets with wire handles were overflowing with plums and peaches, glistening like dark jewels under the old lights. We were enlisted in putting fresh oilcloth on the shelves, ready to receive the Ball jars. *Clostridium botulinum* had no chance against the women as they inspected the fruits and vegetables for blemishes. The jar rubbers, lids, racks, containers of sugar and utensils were sterilized and prepared for the fresh, firm fruit. It was almost a minuet as Helen and Sophie moved gracefully back and forth between the stove and the tables.

I remember the colors of the beets and carrots and the pale pink of the crabapple jelly and the laughter as the women engaged in a passionate pickling of cucumbers, carefully lining the old crocks with horseradish leaves.

I'll keep my fax and modem, program my VCR, and wear my estrogen patch, but something is irrevocably lost. We are all somehow diminished when a culture changes. In the meantime, I will keep clipping recipes, buying thread, and collecting Ball jars just in case.

P.S. Ball announced on August 25, 1992, they were not canning the canning business.

September 1992

Cows
in the Belfrey

Many Americans have fantasies about another career, especially busy executives. A quaint little bookstore, perhaps? A charming, oh-so-chic restaurant, an antique store, upscale, trendy, American Primitive, 18th century French, 19th century English or Art Deco, or a bed and breakfast inn. I had the same vision. To live among polished antiques and fresh flowers from the garden, to have interesting and witty guests with whom to share a bon mot, to dabble in the culinary arts, and have the same cultured and refined guests applaud and shout "Brava, encore, bellissima."

Why did I want to own an inn? Eight years of watching Bob Newhart shows. Far too many reruns of Bing Crosby and Danny Kaye in *Holiday Inn*. Two solid years of life on the Continent. Months of ecstasy in Italy, lazy wine-soaked days of life on the cheap in a pensione, discussing art and history far into the Roman night. Many trips to England, Wales, and Scotland. A grandmother who was a caterer. A brother who was a chef and whose business mentor was the great Mr. Stouffer himself. It was in my genes. The Poles for centuries had a reputation for hospitality, a country flat as a pancake and open to any and all invaders.

I was going to get out from behind that keyboard and live my dream. And I did. Answered prayers, as it were. Do be careful or you will get what you pray for.

We searched New Hampshire, Maine, and Vermont for an old Victorian house which we would lovingly restore. This was the '80s. Everyone was in a feeding frenzy in real estate. It was now or never. I found my house through *Yankee Magazine.* I compared it to a beautiful woman who needed the right makeup and jewels, nothing major, just some cosmetic changes. Lighting, landscaping, a new driveway, a new roof, new gutters, new porches, nothing major, a good cleaning and scrubbing, replace broken windows, buy furniture, buy appliances, buy antiques, buy curtains, hire various trades, nothing major, have the floors sanded and polished (crew of four for three weeks), choose wallpapers, hire wallpaper hangers, have the antique registers scraped and repainted, hire housepainters (crew of six for three months) to scrape and paint. Nothing major.

Create the logo, create a name, obtain a trademark. People think that Amberwood has some mystical connection to Poland. Actually, it is named after my golden retriever, Marshall's Amber Lady, age 12. Polish amber is exquisite and there are several grades, but it has nothing to do with the inn. Find some angle, some shtick. Just like the burlesque queens in the musical *Gypsy*, ya gotta have a gimmick. I took all the endings from British names, and matched them with prefixes like Stonecroft, Ferncroft, Ambercroft, Stonewood, Applewood, Maplewood.

Market nationally to more than 12 million Americans of Polish descent. Revive all my old academic connections, American Historical Association, American Association for the Advancement of Slavic Studies, lovingly called AAASS.

So I bought the house on a Sunday. This is an important point in my tale. Never buy any piece of property on a Sunday. Not in a village. Not on land that faces the Post Office. Not in an area where the mail is not so much delivered as picked up. In cars. And trucks. With doors slamming.

Instead of reading all those books about how to start an inn, I estimated costs by the 100-day rule that says take the number of rooms you have, multiply by the amount you can make each night in all those rooms, and multiple by 100, so I was looking at a $15,000 to $20,000 gross income. This was going to be wonderful. I would have a gift shop. I would do lunches-to-go for people weary of fast food. I would go to crochet class and sit on the porch and crochet and wait for guests. I would play the piano. I would be dead wrong.

Instead of reading all those books, I should have read Shirley Jackson's story, "The Lottery." I should have read every book that Stephen King ever wrote. And I should have read more about the peculiar tri-county area of north-eastern Vermont known as the Northeast Kingdom.

Writer Leland Kinsey calls the Northeast Kingdom a slightly presumptuous but accurate name for this somewhat distant and difficult-to-live-in quarter of Vermont. This is not a place one eases into, or where one lives by accident, or just happens to be. One lives here by birth or choice, probably both, and it is an ongoing decision. Twelve percent unemployment. A place where most of the phone book has five last names in it. (Did you see *Deliverance?*) Major industry—logging, dairy farming, tourism. A state said to have more cows than people in it. That is a myth. They just prefer it that way.

Canada is fifteen miles away. Montreal is two hours to the north, and Montreal is warmer. The winters are brutal; 30 below is nothing on my porch. The winds come howling through with a vengeance and I look outside at drifts three feet high and have anxiety attacks, thinking what would happen if I needed a doctor or a hospital. How cold was it? It was so cold that I never knew if I was having hot flashes or too many cats were sleeping on the bed. You have heard of three-dog nights. Well, we had a lot of cats.

Spring is brief. About a week. Mud season is a very real season. Forsythia and rhododendrons and roses won't grow here. We are halfway between the Equator and the North Pole, but we are in the mountains so it is colder. Our leaves are usually out by May 10 and they fall down by October 10. We are inundated by leaf peepers during foliage season and, of course, phone calls asking us when exactly the leaves were turning.

Boston is consistently 10-20 degrees warmer, ditto New York; we are four hours from Boston and six from New York. No one works on the first day of hunting season or the first day of trout fishing or during the county fair. There is a different rhythm of life in the North Country. People work the ski industry as maids and waiters, then the snow melts and they collect unemployment. So much for the cheap labor pool.

Stuart and I have a handyman named Dick, who has worked for us the past three years. He is deaf and Stuart is deaf, so they scream at each other and tell tall tales and have a great time. They are contemporaries and both served in World War II. I have heard the same stories thousands of times. Both men are good carpenters and terrible at washing windows.

The housekeeper is a local woman who is conscientious and a hard worker. They lost the dairy farm and it almost killed her husband. She works with us in the daytime and more hours for spring cleaning and fall cleaning. She has four sisters in the area and three grown children. I figure I better watch myself, because if I rile her up, we will alienate 32% of the local population with her family alone.

When we had an Easter Open House and invited 85 people, we hired four people to work as bartender and servers. They had never seen puff pastry. They were afraid of the caviar. They had never seen an Easter egg tree. If you need four people to work a special event, hire eight. Four usually won't show.

There are wonderful native Vermonters, people who are kind but nonetheless very reserved. Hardworking, civic-minded Vermonters. And there is a dark side to Vermont, an underculture, where women and animals and children are nothing more than property, where education is despised, and outsiders feared and hated.

I had no idea the village had no police protection. You could call the state troopers but they were an hour away at best. I thought we could get cable TV. Wrong again. We pay $11.21 a month to get the basic three networks, public television, Chicago, and Grand Old Opry.

Living in Boston most of my life, I am basically outgoing and direct. Stu and I are the most nonthreatening couple in the world. I am a middle-aged, overweight woman who wears glasses. Stuart is twenty-five years older than I am, a retired professor, white hair, glasses, with an authentic New England accent. He was reared 45 minutes from Barton, Vermont, the son and grandson of farmers. What a pair we are, fat and old and nice. Were people smirking at us? Was it just our imagination?

Why were people trespassing on our property and giving us a very quaint sign with their finger? What sort of language did they speak, native Vermontese perhaps? As one sullen young lad put it, "We have the right to walk here. Go back where you came from, flatlander." At least the people in Maine called those not born there "from away." Not in Vermont. We are *flatlanders*. They have T-shirts that say "Native Vermont and proud of it" on the anterior, and the posterior reads, "Flatlander, go home."

We learned other new words. *Wigwags*—that's a railroad signal. We have the Canadian Pacific Railroad on our property line. And *blow-offs*. Not what you think. It has to do with a system of running water all winter so your pipes don't freeze. And *springers.* Has to do with cattle.

We had to stay at a motel in Barton while the varnished floors were drying. There was a calf bellowing outside. Stuart left, then came back, and I asked him what happened. "Oh," he said, "I had to drive the calf back across the road." I stupidly asked, "How did you fit him into the car?"

I also made points with the local farmer who raises succulent pheasants for the restaurant market by complimenting him on his chickens. And we managed to rile up the whole town over what we and our lawyer called a private nuisance and they called a sacred tradition. One Monday before Christmas at 9 a.m., I was blasted out of bed by "Jingle Bell Rock" playing outside my window. Because we are on a hill, sound travels up in the cold air. Following that ditty were "Frosty the Snowman" and "Alvin and the Chipmunks."

I am not a morning person. I probably should do BED AND LUNCH, not bed and breakfast. Stuart says, "Did you get up on the wrong side of the web this morning?" I made some phone calls and found out the music was coming from the loudspeakers pointed at our house, on top of a building, privately owned, by the Chamber of Commerce. The Chamber of Commerce we had just joined. We had attended our first meeting and only one person said hello to us.

The president of the Chamber of Commerce slogged up our long steep driveway to tell us that they were not allowed to play religious music, as someone had objected to it, so their cassette of the aforementioned music would be played from 9 a.m. to 5 p.m., six days a week, for the two full weeks before Christmas. We protested. Our lawyer protested. They said no one had ever complained. We said the previous owner was stone deaf for years and then the house was vacant; of course, no one ever complained. Then the man who insured both our cars and all our property wrote a letter to the local paper saying we should go back where we came from; how dare we flatlanders tell the village what to do. Hate mail started coming in—illiterate hate mail. Anonymous phone calls. More letters to the editor. We remained silent. We changed insurance agents. No one spoke to us. We had lived there less than eight weeks.

This provided the perfect introduction to the zoning board—those sage citizens who all looked like Larry, Darryl, and Darryl. My neighbor, who owns the Barton Inn, is an entrepreneur with a restaurant background. We are the same age; she is Greek-American and I am Polish-American. She came to Barton from Boston a year earlier than we had and renovated the place she bought. "No matter what the zoning board says, no matter how ridiculous, do not lose your temper," she advised. She sat behind me during the meeting, and as the questions were asked, she poked me in the back.

"What kinda people zactly you folks reckon your place will bring in to our village?" I wanted to say, all the folks you hate, all the colors, all the religions—"

"You don't have enough parking. Let's get out the rule books."

"How can you be open all year?" I pointed out that the Northeast Kingdom was a twelve-month resort. They didn't understand what that was. Reluctantly, they gave us the zoning permit. By the way, the property is zoned commercial. And when I looked at the zoning chairperson, he had colder eyes than I have seen in an aquarium.

I was soaking wet with sweat when we got out of there. My neighbor said I showed remarkable restraint for a hot-headed, pig-headed Polack. And indeed I had.

After the zoning board meeting came the unannounced visit of the State Health Inspector. She went through each drawer, under all the beds, in all the china cabinets, through all the silverware, and ran her gloved finger around the toilets. We needed thermometers in the refrigerators.

We got our rating sheet and our restaurant license and lodging license. The state makes visits about twice a year, always unannounced and usually after some disaster in cleanliness has just occurred—the puppy wet on the floor as I was carrying him from his crate, Stu left a coffee cup in the microwave. All in all, she was tough but fair. I learned to never mess with the State.

Never mess with a moose either. If you think you see a tall man in a brown suit on the road waving his arms at you, it is probably a moose. Stop the car and slowly back away, even if you hit another car. Your rate of survival will be better than if you just stand there or try to go forward. DO NOT BLOW YOUR HORN. The moose will charge and demolish your car, or try to make love to it, which for a 1700-pound bull moose is about the same thing.

We mingled with the flora and fauna of the Northeast Kingdom. If you are driving near Barton and you have managed not to hit any of the deer that bounded in front of you, and you hear the slapping of bare feet near your car, move away cautiously. I thought it odd that a barefooted man would be on I-91 at night, a very HAIRY barefooted man, then realized it was huge bear crossing the road. On a spring night, you can sit on the porch and watch the processions of skunks, mama and all the babies, in single file, proceed from under the front porch of the Barton Inn and move slowly down the sidewalk and across the street. We had a white rabbit who lived on our property in the storage house for a whole year.

Besides our handyman and the housekeeper, we have trash haulers. For three years, their truck has been coming up the steep drive on Saturday at noon. I sent Christmas and Easter cards to Mr. and Mrs. Poulin and the children. I always said hello at the Grand Union supermarket and the church bazaar.

I asked my neighbor if she sent cards to the trash-hauling couple. "What? They are not married." "So what?" I said. "You have been addressing cards to Mr. and Mrs. all this time?" "Yes." She started to laugh uproariously. "Not only are they not married," she said. "He is not a he, he is a she. Didn't you know? Her name is a woman's name." I said, "Oh, no, I thought it was a French name similar to Leslie and Leslie or Chris and Chris." Oh, well, I erred on the side of the angels, so to speak. And I don't care. We get along and that's fine with me.

Just as I want the government and the church to stay out of my underpants, so we stay out of the guests' underpants. Remember the days when it was illegal to register as man and wife if you weren't married? Not any more. We never, never ask. Have the guests sign the register. Never assume who is married, who is single, various genders or kinships, significant others. We never say, "How is your father, dear?" "That's not my father, that is my husband." (Stu and I go through this all the time.)

I have no horror stories for you. The innkeepers get together every once in a while and tell some frightening tales. Things stolen or damaged. Knock on wood; we have never had anything taken or broken. I was very paranoid in the beginning but now I just say to myself, "If they want to steal, they will." The only thing ever verifiably missing was six toothbrushes from the guest bathroom, which are there for guests' use. The only people in the house that night were a pair of dentists, but we can't prove they did it.

We really don't care who sleeps with whom and we believe that groceries in the bedroom can be a source of entertainment or even a source of inspiration. In the creative foodstuff area, I suppose, whipped cream comes readily to mind. But we did have a couple who left puddles of maple syrup in the boudoir. While I have learned that who washes the sheets knows all, I figure if it comes out, who cares? We are still trying to figure out how the maple syrup got on the ceiling.

I felt like Bette Midler, who said of Madonna, "I would hate to be the maid that rinses out those delicates."

Whatever you have been through in your career in business, working in the hospitality business where one deals with bodily functions on a daily basis is a true window to the world. Romance knows no age limits. Our most energetic and insatiable guests are usually a bit long in the tooth. After the ardor cools in a twenty- or thirty-year marriage, it is not uncommon for travel and new places to act as an aphrodisiac. All the doors lock from the inside with hooks. I find people reluctant to use them and there are often surprise entries on the guest floor. There is more than just sap running on my property in the spring when the days are warm and the nights are cool. We have no telephones or televisions in the guest rooms and try to provide a contemplative atmosphere, and if the guests choose to contemplate one another, I am very happy.

We had some guests who were there for a wedding. The night was quiet but in the morning, all the shrubbery was festooned with condoms. I don't know how they got the screens out, or why they did what they did, but everyone going to Father Roy's early Sunday mass got a good look at our bushes. We never said a word; we just pretended we were picking raspberries.

When questioned, the late great hostess Perle Mesta was asked why her parties were so successful. She answered, "Oh, hell, honey, I just give them whiskey and peanuts." I was an admirer of hers.

My philosophy is to give the guests what I would want, which is usually to be left alone, no chitchat, no questions. If a guest wants to chat, we are happy to talk. A nice bed with sheets that have been washed and hung outside and ironed. Big thick towels and washcloths. Decent soap. Lots of Kleenex. Good toilet paper. A large glass of orange juice. Homemade food, plenty of it. Bottled water, wine coolers, soft drinks, lots of ice. And a sense of a safe harbor. Not just women traveling alone, but men and couples too. It is a dangerous world out there. They can leave expensive camera equipment or merchandise in the room and lock it. We are here and no one will touch their belongings. We go to bed when the last guest is in, no matter how late. We accept no guest off the street, if our guests are already sleeping.

When you come to an old-fashioned B&B, you become part of the family. I have washed the bathing suits of a family of four—a law professor from Georgetown and his lovely wife and two teenage children. I washed the clothes of two military men who were traveling from Eastern Canada on a motorcycle and got caught in a terrible storm. They sat around in two of my frilly bathrobes and drank milk, by the way, and we made them supper, no charge. They couldn't go out; they had no change of clothes.

People blown in by storms, terrified by the power of nature and usually having no inkling of the geography, have provided us with some of our nicest evenings, as we fed them homemade onion soup, turkey sandwiches, lemon cake, and a bottle of wine.

We made mistakes, too, like not counting the family cats and leaving Charlotte Marie in the pink room. The couple went to bed, and Charlotte shot out from underneath the bed. The woman saw in the darkness only black and white and decided there was a skunk in the room and she screamed and fell out of the bed. Her husband started laughing. The other guests heard this, and soon they all were up and laughing. Close call for us. Close call for Charlotte Marie.

One night we were asleep downstairs, with a full house upstairs. I thought I heard Emily Louise, sister cat to

Charlotte, playing with a new squeaky toy. Wait a minute, we didn't buy the cat a new squeaky toy. Emily was playing with a bat. As I was screaming and Stuart was stuffing an apron in my mouth, the bat was flying all around. Finally by turning on all the lights and shooing the bat out, we again went to sleep. You guessed it. Bat number two started swooping around. I did a lot of screaming that night.

Two delightful French ladies wanted to run the hydrobath and got all gussied up in their bathcaps and jammies, but the bath wouldn't work. I came up and fooled with it and said, "Oh, some frog must have gotten stuck in it." As soon as I said it, I knew that *frog* was not the best choice of words on my part. "Pairhaps, one of our countrymen got, how you zay, stuck, n'est-ce pas?" she said.

I also locked out a guest and went to bed. Not just any guest. The principal of the local school.

We get to practice medicine too. The innkeeper as doctor treats insomnia, backache, dizziness, headache, and bun-ache (cyclists), fever, sunburn, cramps, sore throat, sniffles, bee-stings, bumps, cuts, scrapes, bruises, monilia, hemorrhoids, arthritis, blisters, rashes, bug bites, constipation, and gas.

I try to do most of my own basic cleaning because in my heart I am a Polish baba and because I am obsessive-compulsive. But like Joan Rivers, I don't work out. I should but I don't. I agree with Joan. If God wanted us to bend over, he'd put diamonds on the floor.

All the guests were nice people. The lady avocado farmer from Australia, the two Spanish engineers, the German couple who stayed a week. The auto mechanic from New Jersey. Three doctors from Michigan who came to us for a cycling vacation; they nearly had coronaries because they were out of shape.

A German couple arrived on July 3 and watched us put the bunting on the house and get ready for the big parade.

They flew into Dorval, an airport in Montreal, and had never been in America alone. They had with them only fifty Canadian dollars and were on their way to Middlebury, Vermont, to visit relatives. We couldn't take their money, so we took their Eurocheck, which cost us a fifteen-dollar fee and a ten-day wait, but I still would not have taken their only cash.

The retired couple, Rosie and Andy. Andy sold his land for a million dollars and they were enjoying spending it. Rosie said to me, "Judith, you and I have a lot in common. We both have a typing business and we both like old men." Yeah, Rosie was right. But *her* old man had a million big ones.

Running a bed and breakfast inn is a happy business, like florists or beauty salons. Occasionally there is a kitchen fire, or Stu cuts his finger so we go to the emergency room twenty miles away. Or as I waltzed out with a large platter ready to take the ten orders of Eggs Benedict, my chef says to me, "All set," and I asked, "Where are the eggs?" Stu had forgotten the eggs.

We had six ladies of the Baptist Church group sitting on the veranda sipping iced tea, when some of the local boys decided to joy-ride naked in a pickup truck with their women. It was romance in the afternoon. It was shocking, horrifying. The women craned their necks and the appropriate comments of outrage were made, when one of the Baptist ladies asked me, "Do you think they will drive by again? I really didn't see all that well."

We had a party of twelve Polish-Americans for a three-day visit. For their first night they had ordered an authentic Polish meal. I had the butcher from Brooklyn order the best beef for the rolls called *zrazy*. Stu took the golden retrievers with him to pick up the beef. The guests arrived and started to play cards. It was 85 degrees. Stuart did not show up and did not call. Three hours later, he called to say the car had broken down and the dogs and he were at a garage, trying to get someone to drive them and the beef back home. We do not have cabs and there are no rental cars. I was wild with frustration and rage. The menu which had been planned for six months was a little late. In four years that was my worst experience, but I learned not to wait until the day of anything.

Then there was the stuffing I made for the turkey, with chestnuts, cognac, onion, celery, spices. I was so proud of myself, but it was disgusting. Stuart said it had no redeeming social value, not even for landfill.

We remember the five Japanese women who rang both doorbells at 4 a.m. They couldn't read the No Vacancy sign.

We remember the Boston attorney who wanted her parents to have an authentic Polish experience and paid for the trip. We prepared the traditional zakaski and iced Polish vodka, the herring, the herbed butter, the marinated mushrooms, the delicate ham, and shrimp appetizers. We brought it to the couple on the porch. The herring in cream and onion is called *sledzie*. "Oh," they said, "What is that?" I explained all the hors d'oeuvres. "Oh, I don't *do* sledzie," he said. "Bring me coffee." Neither the man nor the woman tried anything. By the way, an expression you might hear in Chicago, where there are more people of Polish descent than in Warsaw, is "tough sledzie."

One Sunday morning we prepared a lovely special breakfast for our two guests, and just as we finished preparing the salmon roulade and just-picked herbs with poached eggs, the fresh fruit cup, and the hot blueberry muffins, the woman rapped on the kitchen door and said, "We are leaving. My husband and I had an argument. Goodbye." I tried to be gracious. I pointed to the hot trays going out to the dining room and said, "Don't feel bad about this." "I won't," she said and left. "Well," I said to Stuart, "Tough sledzie." We went into the dining room, sat down, and enjoyed a marvelous breakfast.

This is a business of instant gratification. They praise the furnishings and ambiance in many languages.

You know, in medical transcription, so often, all we hear is complaints. Maybe that is why I like the hospitality business so much. Also, we do not wait to be paid.

On a Sunday morning six or eight people sit down together. Perhaps they are shy. They may speak two or even three languages in the dining room. They make tentative approaches to each other. The silver, the crystal, the china, the fresh flowers, the candles. The music, Chopin perhaps or Scott Joplin, Verdi or Puccini. The guests are rested, they are relaxed. They are breathing mountain air.

The glorious maples in front of the house form a cathedral of color, green in the summer, crimson-gold in the fall. The white wicker, the huge baskets of red geraniums, the sensuous exotic fuchsia, the hummingbirds. Champagne corks pop, fresh honeydew melon is waiting, with raspberries picked in my yard that morning, a light creme sauce, fresh pineapple.

The next course is served. The guests have popovers, jam, mushroom and ham omelettes, home fries, pierogi, kielbasa from my Cleveland butcher, homemade makowiec, poppyseed roll and strawberry cookies, and move on to coffee and liqueurs, Grand Marnier, creme de menthe. We offer, they taste. They now are more relaxed and become more expansive, willing to part with more of themselves and more of their life experience. The *New York Times* and *Boston Globe* arrive and they move to the veranda. The young man from Israel, the old couple from Peoria, the antique dealer from Montreal and his wife. They are understanding their differences and their similarities.

Stu and I shut the big door to the dining room, make sure the candles are out, and begin to clear the dishes. What a business.

Note: Amberwood operated for five years. Judith Marshall left Barton on February 21, 1993, for a position in Greater Boston. The inn is empty and dark and for sale.

Under My Babushka

The medical transcription business was supposed to be recession-proof. I was counting on full beds everywhere. Now I hear the census is down. People are putting off elective surgery. People cannot pay the co-payment. People have lost their health insurance. They are not going to the doctor or the hospital. The health information managers (HIMs) are sitting on their wallets. They are not so quick to call for overload transcription help.

HIMs are getting smarter too. They ask for a software count with a bill. They ask more questions. They demand quality and turnaround and they want to pay less for it. Not more. Less. People are dealing, and bids I hear sound like 1971 bids, not 1992.

And keep it up, AHIMA members. It is about time you knew how to count or look at a by-the-page charge and see that there were two-sentence paragraphs. Or that a byte is not a character. Or the difference between a well-established ethical firm and a here-today, gone-tomorrow outfit.

The transcription industry is evolving at the speed of light. Some hospitals are going under. Others are consolidating. The little neighborhood facility is now a satellite clinic or an office building. Transcription services are merging. Digital dictation is everywhere. Electronic transmission of data is changing work patterns for millions of people. Where are you, Studs Terkel?

I called AT&T and New England Telephone about getting an 800 number for a digital system. "Do you wish to have intrastate service, only Vermont, or do you wish to service the northern hemisphere?" Well, golly, I want the northern hemisphere. The English-speaking world is my oyster.

There is a new type of owner and a new type of worker. There are venture capitalists with bags of money and a stable of keyboarding fillies and a digital capacity out the wazoo.

When someone tells me they are driving around the countryside picking up tapes and delivering work, they must be a small outfit with a doctor client base. The rest of us are uploading, downloading, modeming, faxing, archiving, compressing, and shrinking to a paperless record from a tapeless digital system.

The workers are changing. They have PCs and medical shorthand software. Every time they type VT for Vermont on a letter, ventricular tachycardia plays out and they don't care. The doctor said, "Lungs are clear." They play out, "The lungs are clear to percussion and auscultation. No rales, wheezes, or rhonchi in either lobe bilaterally." You can Betadine your sweet aspidistra, they are paid on production. Remind me to toggle off PRD+ when I am writing abortion issues. About issues, sorry.

Aspiring transcriptionists sometimes take a correspondence course and they have a medical dictionary on hard drive and they are in business. Some call themselves *CMTs* because their school or their course sent them a certificate of completion (and they think a certificate means they are certified). And you can't see what they look like because they live three states away; all you know is their voice. And all they know, Mr. Employer, is your voice. The workday is now

24 hours long and three time zones long. Nine to five is dead.

They read all the computer magazines but don't belong to a professional society. They never worked in a hospital. There is no ongoing ethics or confidentiality training. Telecommuting has created an incredible, zany, ridiculous kaleidoscope of people, with an in-yer-face attitude, with total fearlessness, who would spit in your eye and swipe your client and sleep like a baby. Many who are hypoferremic in character are drawn to a computerized business, where personal accountability is often distant and anonymous.

This is not at all bad. Let the floodgates open and let a whole new fresh and bright group of wannabes try their luck. When I am swilling down Mylanta and adjusting my Estraderm patch, I am eager to work with keyboard-literate hotshots and I want men to come aboard (because wages will rise). I want the smell of aftershave to permeate my mornings at AHIMA or AAMT or MTIA (Medical Transcription Industry Alliance) meetings.

With MTIA membership restricted to those grossing more than half a million a year (later this was changed to a hundred thousand dollars a year), I daresay the smell of money will also waft about the meeting hall. While we expected hospitals to become megacorporations, did we really expect the business of transcription to be fragmented in some lithotripsy of supply and demand? Should a hospital with constant overload dissect its 10,000 lines a day into five different small services? (Some do this because they don't want to "put all their eggs in one basket." For cryin' out loud.)

Who will speak for transcriptionists now? The combined membership of MTIA will control and affect the lives of more MTs than AAMT's 9,000 membership. Will an organization evolve for the solo practitioners or the small-potatoes club of less than $100,000 gross?

Is the business of AAMT really business? Until recently, it was not. In the bad old days, we would try to discuss prices or wages and someone would start screaming about the Sherman Antitrust Act. This year, it cost extra money to attend the special Business Issues section at the Annual Meeting. Does that mean AAMT really wants to represent only MTs who work in hospitals? Or does this new section just open up a new market possibility and increased revenues for AAMT? Founded for the purposes of education and certification, does the Association essentially serve all its members in those capacities?

Anyone who was worried the transcriptionists would unionize back in the formation period of 1978-1982 can now relax. It seems we are being polarized and more compartmentalized, as in the Business Issues section. How many transcriptionists are there, anyway? Estimates were 50,000 many years ago. I always thought that was a very low figure.

Who will promote AMA recognition for medical transcriptionists? Will AAMT membership rise? How exactly will MTIA and AHIMA focus on issues in the workplace, productivity measurement, pricing, education, and confidentiality? MTIA and AHIMA both represent employers, of course.

No answers under my babushka, only questions.

October 1992

No Flies on Me

Rollin', rollin', rollin', keep them dogies rollin', rawhide!
Don't bother me today. I have a million lines to type on my sophisticated system. I must include job numbers, tape numbers, dictation numbers, line counts, character counts, software verification sheets, payroll sheets, time in, time out, hours of work, and give double coupons on Tuesdays. They want logs with full patient names, attending physician names, resident names, intern names, admission dates, discharge dates, consultation dates, and creation of a file for each patient. They want a call at 7:30 a.m. before we modem so they can watch the printout. I can't modem when I wanna.

We are so busy adjusting, accommodating, bending, correcting, circumventing, fixing, smoothing over, counting with software, counting without software, and somehow trying to make a buck. The money is down, energy costs are up, and it is kiss-kiss because competition is chopping prices.

Three women in the past week who live here, in rural poverty on a mountain, want to make at least ten dollars an hour with full benefits and Vermont Blue Cross. They don't know the first thing about medical transcription. They want me to supply the computers, books, training, transcribers, and the work. They had the idea somehow that the medical industry is waiting for them with boxes of tapes and they have a week or two to transcribe them. They don't need Gloria Steinem. Their self-esteem is tippy-top. It's mine that needs a transfusion.

We are between a rock and a rock: technology to speed things up and the relentless drive for total quality demanded by the health information managers, quality that requires thought and time. But the source of the transcription is the dictation; dictation practices which are cost-INeffective can and must be changed. We transcriptionists have honed our skills despite an explosion of information and terminology and mastered computer skills.

Dictating doctors still whisper, chew gum, eat lunch, or just are incredibly bad and no one corrects them. They never learn to hold the microphone or the telephone. They never learn they are in America now and the patient is Robert Smith, not Smith Robert. And Lord help us, why are we forever plagued with doctors with colds and terrible sinus conditions whispering all those Ob-Gyn procedures and pediatric summaries, with quiet little annoying voices? Speak up, fill your lungs with air, and talk to me plainly and loudly. Be delicate and subservient at home or wherever you came from, but here, kiddo, when you dictate, *belt it out!*

Transcriptionists are so flexible, our spines are like pasta. But the docs go marching on, oblivious to any criticism or questions or kindly suggestions. Why are they allowed to repeat lengthy histories and physicals on discharge summaries when those records are already in the chart?

Pertinent positives and negatives never went out of style. Why, in this age of macros and medical word expanders, are physicians dictating cataract surgery, the D&C, tonsillectomy, laparoscopic cholecystectomy, and total abdominal hysterectomy over and over when many are exactly the same every time? Are HIMs encouraging physicians to offer their standard surgical notes for a macro?

If a patient is deceased, God rest his soul, is it really necessary in cases of elderly people with multisystem disease for the doctor to dictate six pages of laboratory data and medication adjustments? Is it necessary to read all nursing notes into the summary on a daily basis? This is not a discharge summary. It is a lazy, stupid, costly exercise on the part of the resident, and the attending who allows it. It teaches little and encourages no real thought on the condition of that patient. In the case of patient transfer, or readmission, the reader must shuffle through and extrapolate meaningful data from a paper blizzard.

We need a lot more templates for endoscopies, for podiatry, dentistry, and obstetrics. With the right approach, many physicians would comply happily and eagerly. A badly dictated newborn summary, adrift in a muddled broth of inches and centimeters and military time, benefits from a rigid and complete format. The nurse/midwives do a quick and efficient job with these; why can't the doctors?

Why are they reading into the record the complete reports of x-rays, exercise tolerance tests, echocardiograms, and pathology reports? And reading them badly, I might add. There are hospitals which have had off-site transcription services doing their work for a decade, yet the physicians dictate as if the transcriptionists are right there on the same floor.

In the dictation they are screaming about their initials not being correct ("I want F.A.S. on my signature, I earned it!"). I have no idea what they are saying. Nothing on my list about it. They know an outside service is doing the work but they persist in giving complex instructions about attaching what to which and looking up addresses. Nothing happens, of course, and they become apoplectic when their orders are ignored. Sometimes I long to pick up the phone and just call him, wherever he is in the United States, and say to his secretary, "Just tell him his work is being done by an off-site service. Let him take up with the hospital how he wants all the attachments and instructions carried out."

Horrible dictation should be nipped in the bud with the same vigor that circumcision is performed on innocent baby boys. No delay. No mercy.

A lot of silliness goes on too. The use of the words "seem" and "appeared." "The patient seemed to be eating better and appeared to be ambulatory without difficulty and was discharged." "The x-ray as interpreted by the radiologist," and "the CBC, with results as interpreted by the laboratory technician," are a trend among younger doctors, abrogating responsibility in every sentence. Pin the error on the donkey or anyone else in the vicinity of the hospital grounds, just in case there is an error.

And the surgeon who says "the patient's blood, the patient's bowel, the patient's femur" all throughout the report. C'mon, who else would be on that table?

All I am saying is, *instead of going faster, why not lighten the load?* Medical transcriptionists are professionals who know dictation best and are never allowed to contribute to its improvement. *It was shut up and type in 1955 and it is shut up and type in 1993.*

We need moral courage from health information managers and transcription supervisors and service owners to go to the source and make effective changes in dictation practices, including real efforts at in-house education.

November 1992

Mrs. Dixon
Goes to Harvard

Once upon a time, there was an older physician who was thoughtful and thorough and who loved his vocation. Each patient was to him more than a set of organs or a disease with a battle plan. His patient was an elderly woman with the sad problems accompanying women of a certain age: heart disease, cataracts, and a little less spring to the step.

I could tell that the doctor respected his patient, Mrs. Dixon, and that he was bound and determined to dictate for her the most complete and dignified expiration summary that he could. He carefully outlined the history of her last illness and he lingered more than usual on the precise and rather literary social histories he was wont to dictate. This was a woman of substance, a woman of means. She was a widow with several children, and I had the impression from this marvelous doctor that she had led a full and contented life and was sensible to the end. She herself had early on in the course of her hospitalization determined that she should have a Do Not Resuscitate status. No bells and whistles for this lady. The horses were turned toward heaven, as they say.

What a privilege and pleasure it is to work for this doctor, and he does not even know me. I don't know him. Only his voice at a large hospital served by my company. But we have a relationship. That is what medical transcription means in the end, a partnership between people like him and people like me serving a patient like her.

I love to transcribe. Each day the slate is wiped clean and I begin again my ramble through the bizarre, the exotic, the mundane, the terrifying and, yes, the disgusting. There are heroes, victims, saviors, innocents, cowards, geniuses, and jerks. . . .

• A surgeon was doing a routine breast biopsy and dropped the scalpel (he said the nurse dropped it), which fell hard on the patient's thigh and lacerated it through the drapes. They sutured the thigh but the patient developed an infection and had to return for an incision and drainage. The breast biopsy was benign. The patient is still fighting sepsis.

• A woman with chronic obstructive pulmonary disease and end-stage emphysema entered a large hospital. She continued to sneak cigarettes, and a cloud of smoke was seen to emanate from her bathroom. She was on nasal oxygen but continued to smoke despite warnings. Now, this woman was a middle-class high school graduate. She should have known that when oxygen meets flame, something happens. But when her male friend came to visit, he sat on the bed and they shared a nip of gin and she asked him to light her cigarette. KABOOM. The explosion killed her, nearly killed him, and blew out the walls. The families sued the hospital, claiming that the hospital was negligent because it failed to warn the patient not to smoke.

• A young mother came in for a breast biopsy after mammographic findings of a lesion. A routine chest x-ray was performed and the patient had a 6 cm unresectable lung carcinoma. She died six months later. She had never smoked a cigarette.

• A scrub nurse is permanently disabled and unable to work. She has an allergy to latex.

• A man was standing on a ladder and pounding nails to put a birdhouse in a tree and he fell off the ladder and landed on a wheelbarrow which rolled down an incline and was hit by a bakery truck. He sustained a fractured leg.

• A woman was sitting in a car in a funeral procession, when the hearse in front of her stopped suddenly and the casket slid out and hit her car. She was thrown forward and backward, hit her head on the dashboard, and sustained a concussion. The funeral was delayed while she was taken by ambulance to a hospital.

• The family of a woman in her nineties came to a famous neurologist's office and told the doctor their mother had fantasies and delusions and hallucinations. She imagined a world of bunny rabbits and elves, fairies, and sprites, vividly colored flowers, babbling brooks and shaded groves with cavorting fawns and ducklings swimming on a lake where it was always summer. The wise doctor counseled the family to take their mother home and prescribed no medication. He told them that her Walt Disney world was harmless and she enjoyed it. No hospitalization, no work-up, no invasive studies, no frightening tests. God bless him.

As for Mrs. Dixon, she had one wish in life, one unfulfilled dream—to attend Harvard University in Cambridge, Massachusetts. So she decided to will her body to science. As the doctor finished his summary, he dictated, "And Mrs. Dixon went to Harvard."

May 1993

It's All Right
to Laugh

It never was a marriage made in heaven. I would tell people he was having a birthday . . . if I let him live. Or that I never thought of divorce. Murder yes, divorce never. All those old vaudeville jokes. Recently I told a friend that my husband and I were like two prehistoric monsters, throttling each other while plunging into an abyss. "What a pretty picture," he said drily.

Many medical transcriptionists go to great lengths to stay out of the medical mill. Maybe we know too much, we hear too much, we understand too much. But I dragged the old goat down to Boston Union Hospital because I wanted to go dancing and he needed a total knee replacement. The internist agreed and ran a routine blood panel, including the relatively new PSA. When the results came back elevated, we paid little attention. When the test was repeated, both of us were sucked into the whirling vortex of healthcare and the business of cancer treatment. We forgot about the dancing.

In Surgery's chilly preop room, I stopped arguing with him long enough to promise I would not let him get chewed up and spit out by that business, sick with chemotherapy, radiation therapy, and radical surgery, only to face a certain demise.

The operative report and the pathology report revealed status post transurethral resection of the prostate, Stage D, with metastases to right pubic ramus.

Feverishly I became an oddsmaker and information machine, carrying around the *Physicians' Desk Reference,* reading medical and surgical tomes and popular magazine articles. One becomes a vessel of ruminative helplessness and devastating vulnerability.

We met with the surgeon, that technically perfect smarmy son-of-a-gun, who alternately pressured and patronized us. He said we should make up our minds in a week. Orchiectomy and Lupron injections were what he could offer us. Leuprolide, the wonder drug of the mid-80's, was expensive, he said, patting his knees thoughtfully. About $600 for each monthly injection. And he would administer it.

"What about diethylstilbestrol?" I piped up. The surgeon-god frowned and asked, "Are you a nurse?" "No," I countered, "I just read a great deal." Here was a man about to sell us the Cadillac of therapy and I had just mentioned a Volkswagen. He admitted he had one or two patients on DES, but the side effects were considerable and it was not his best recommendation.

We began the trek for another opinion, but not before I was hyperventilating into a paper bag, screaming about the cost of what I called the $600 erection. That is what Lupron does. It allows for an erection. So the Blue Cross folks get the Lupron and the Medicare-without-supplement group gets DES. And everyone gets an orchiectomy.

We saw a kind oncologist. At least he asked about our marriage and our hobbies, which at this point were dwindling rapidly. We asked for better odds and got none. But it was worth the time to speak with someone who had no vested interest in our decision. My stoic husband sat impassively through these interviews, like a sleepy toad on a rock. I thought he was not even paying attention. But he was. He reminded me that only 30% of patients receiving orchiectomy are alive at the end of three years. That meant 70% were dead.

The Veterans Administration told my husband (captain in the U.S. Army for five years, overseas, during World War II) he was not eligible for Lupron there because our income is more than $23,000. "Don't worry," I said to Stu. "Take the DES and we'll go through hot flashes together, and I can lend you the underwear for the gynecomastia. We can both feel like a blast furnace and save on the heating bill."

He developed other symptoms. His medication was changed in the hospital, and he developed shortness of breath and swollen ankles. I urged him to call his internist and tell him. "I am out of shape," he said, "just a bit winded." "You need Lasix," I said. He demurred and he suffered. Heartless and cruel that I am, off I went to bingo. "Call 911 if you get worse. I am going out." He did call his doctor, who told him to relax and called in a prescription to our pharmacy. Xanax. The doctor prescribed an antianxiety agent. More screaming from me, but I took my husband's Xanax and I was fine. He again visited his internist and came out with Lasix, of course.

Truly, I have no magical bag of tricks as a medical language specialist. Not even Wonder Woman can ward off all these bullets with her bracelets. But I will see to it he does not become like my Uncle Ralph, a devastated man after castration, who put on his bathrobe and never left his house again. Women really do handle some things much better. We literally hand over a breast or a uterus, have our surgery, get cured or not, put on our suits or our aprons, and go back to work.

Well, the Bickersons called a truce and decided to have as much fun as possible. Maybe April in Paris, or limping around the dance floor, movies, candlelit dinners, friends, family, golden retrievers, pinochle, fishing, books, whatever we can do each day to feel good. Hillary and Bill and the great American move to national healthcare came a little late for us. We will take one day at a time, enjoy life as much as possible, and he will die with his orchids on.

October 1993

Killing Fleas
with Howitzers

An old Swahili or Hindu blessing is "May this house be safe from tigers." Appropriate for Africa or India but hardly Michigan or Southern California.

Robert L. Love, a Houston attorney writing in the *Journal of the American Association for Medical Transcription*, sees danger from tigers everywhere. This self-styled expert on the medical record seeks to scare the average transcriptionist into purchasing malpractice insurance, and rails against the electronic signature. The attorney also received quite a bit of publicity in *For the Record* a few weeks ago, warning MTs who owned property they may lose it if they are not insured for malpractice.

In a staccato style best left to the writers on *Saturday Night Live*, Love posits himself as savior and seer. Has this guy ever listened to foreign residents dictating operative notes? They are not worried about malpractice or murder of the English language, if indeed that is what they are speaking. What history or precedent has ever taken place in the United States that would make MTs take this sort of fright tactic seriously? Does Love have a kickback arrangement with the insurance industry? Most insurance companies don't even know what insurance this is he is recommending. And why is a professional association for medical transcriptionists listening to this fellow?

103

Hot topics in the literature today are the electronic signature, verbatim transcription, the computerized medical record, and now, liability insurance for MTs. To me, they are all related to one thing—the abrogation by physicians of responsibility for the work they do.

Instead of preparing ourselves for the computerized medical record and recognizing the electronic signature for what it is—a tool to achieve a goal of organization and speed—we are going off in scattered directions on expensive, needless tangents. In 1958 the radiology department where I worked had rubber stamps made with the doctors' signatures. They dictated, we transcribed, and a clerk affixed a rubber stamp signature to each report. No big deal then. No big deal now.

When I transcribe, I am in a partnership with the physician. Both of us bring skill and expertise to the finished document, and the physician's signature verifies his or her responsibility for the report. I cannot control what the doctor, the hospital, Joint Commission, and AHIMA do. I can control only what I do.

To exhort MTs to purchase malpractice insurance is ludicrous, absolutely ridiculous, without any history in the courts. I resent it when a hotshot lawyer tries to scare my colleagues, most of whom are not college graduates and who are still wont to believe Love's arrogance and air of superiority. I think he is dangerous because he is getting a lot of play in the literature and because it looks as if my professional association supports his views.

I disagree that errors and omissions insurance is necessary for the hospital-based or the independent, or that it is a cost of doing business. I would hope that MTs who are self-employed, who own their own businesses and employ other MTs, and most especially members of MTIA reply vociferously to this guru and tell him he is peddling bunk.

We are on the precipice of a new era in healthcare in this country. AHIMA, AAMT, and MTIA working with JCAHO will create new pathways in medical records never before imagined.

The medical transcriptionist, the average medical transcriptionist, is underpaid, part of a secretarial pool, and classified by the government as a clerk-typist. I want AAMT to deal with that, not create an environment of fear where some sort of mythical insurance is required so that we can work.

I want MTIA to deal with Robert Love and his ilk. I don't want parasites on my fringe, pontificating about matters of which they know not. I want accountability of the physicians when they dictate. Plain and clear.

For myself, I don't worry. As a business owner or as transcription supervisor for an old, well-established corporation plugged into every conceivable legal requirement, I am all right. What sends my hackles rising is the ignorant, misdirected advice of a man with a mission. Fanatics of any kind warrant my attention.

What scares me is that MTs are reading what this man advocates. What scares me is that they believe his half-baked nonsense. What scares me is that we are supposed to be the patsies for the almighty doctors.

We are all of us now engaged in a struggle to control costs, to deliver a product faster and better, despite the monumental stupidity of many dictators.

We want to encourage young people, men and women, to enter our field. What is the average wage paid by a hospital? What is required to enter the field? How much does it cost to belong to the local, regional, and national AAMT? Where are our priorities? Is someone making $8.60 an hour at a hospital supposed to go out and buy medical malpractice insurance?

We have more foreign residents in our hospitals than ever before in our history, and some lawyer is telling me that

I have to pay for insurance for the privilege of doing this dictation? I will tell my students that when they get a job at $9.00 an hour in a local hospital, they will be paying $100 per year for membership in AAMT and, of course, their malpractice insurance. The students will hoot me out of the room.

Show me a case where a medical transcriptionist was involved in malpractice. Tell me how to add the cost of this insurance to my fee and why any hospital would pay it. Help me understand why the graying of the industry work force perturbs me and how a meeting of my local chapter is a blur of older women discussing their grandchildren, their retirement, and their bodily deterioration.

I saw the film *Jurassic Park* and noted the first killing by the prehistoric monsters was the lawyer, while he sat on a toilet, having abandoned his charges. Lawyer-bashing is fashionable, no doubt, given the jokes about sharks and lawyers, but sometimes understandable when confronted with Mr. Love aiming his howitzer.

November 1993

Bigeminy Cricket
and Other Ravings

We have endured a severe New England winter by the integument of our teeth, but the laughs were never far away. After five years in Vermont and now 13 months in a Boston medical transcription company, I can tell you unequivocally that working in an office can make you just as crazy as working alone.

We have a physician who never uses the last syllable of a word and gives the sentence ending as *pert* for *period*. I met several women who do his dictation pert. I am starting to talk like him pert. I think I even understand him pert. I probably even like him pert. Isn't he just a tiny bit repetitive pert. But he is better than Dr. David Chin with a Chinese name who speaks Mexican Spanishly pert.

We also have a psychiatrist with a lisp who does the same thing, ending the sentence with a *pewiod*. One gets used to this pewiod. He has a patient who thinks she looks like an ant dressed up with a feather in her hat pewiod. She probably does pewiod. I don't care anymore pewiod. Quality control was never popular but is more necessary than ever pewiod.

What Did You Say, Doctor?

Operative scar on the back of the spine. He was placed on a diet of NPO.

Pain in the left fifth toe, right foot.

She was discharged home with VNA services in hand.

Condition on discharge: In the pink.

Condition on discharge: This woman is on thin ice.

Condition on discharge: His general condition took a nosedive.

Chief complaint: "I don't need a doctor. I am a doctor."

Chief complaint: Liver and onions.

Chief complaint: His arm swelled to humungous proportions. This was in large measure due to its very small size.

The patient looked older than she appeared.

There was a bowling-ball-like texture, indicating an enormous fecal impaction. Disimpaction removed some but this was just the tip of the iceberg.

Due to the levity of his situation, Do Not Resuscitate status was discussed.

She was the first of two twins.

He has chronic anemia; it sits around a hematocrit of 35.

The patient had a leg amputation on the left-hand side.

She will be discharged on her usual medication and Florinef and what have you.

He had been admitted to rule out MI but it didn't pan out.

The patient does not smoke but he sure enjoys his liquor.

The patient needs fine tuning of several medical problems.

Condition on discharge: The patient perked up.

Preoperatively noted was a right inguinal hernia, unfortunately, which he refused to have repaired, reared its head, during his postop stay.

An 83-year-old white male, status post penile implant seven years ago. He must be a fun sort of guy.

The patient lives at home with his wife and a portion of his children.

Condition on discharge: Swell.

A hemicolectomy was performed for what appeared to be an obvious carcinoma.

The patient had substantial narcotic usage during her hospital stay and received 75 mg of Demerol q.3h. on the nose.

The pericardial disease appeared to be a red herring.

Following antibiotic therapy, the patient's pain defervesced rapidly.

I have a discharge summary here on Geraldine Croake. She did.

The Physician as Poet

The nerve root was markedly flattened, almost to ribbons, and discolored a pinkish hue.

ESL Dictation

The patient's general condition went down the hill.

He had an accelerated temperature.

We did a stool for ovary and parasites.

She had boots of nausea.

The patient complained of leg and cow pain.

He had no fever, nausea, or chillies.

Chief complaint: Lack of spirit.

Hello, Risk Management?

The patient has marginal intelligence and minimal common sense.

The nurses assisted the patient in her narcotic addiction by giving her too much pain medication.

Discharge orders: Hold Adriamycin in light of recent radiation.

New Transcriptionist

Seasonal allergy to *Poland* (pollen).

He had a lot of *waterbowl* wheezing (audible).

Studies were consistent with a *secretary* endometrium (secretory).

We just had time for a *kosher* examination of the esophagus (cursory).

She was a *Presbyterian* white female (depressed-appearing).

The patient suffered from *Syracuse vines* in the legs (varicose veins).

Marshall Law for Transcription Owners
The smaller the account, the bigger the aggravation.

The more you need the check, the longer you will wait.

The new employee, whose references were not checked, has a record, is pregnant, and drinks on the job.

April 1994

Lost on the Information Highway

Adapted from a speech to business executives at the Fifth Annual Conference of Medical Transcription Services in New Orleans on April 29, 1994.

I am glad I'm getting you first before the humidity and the mint juleps take their toll.

It is not easy for me, the frequently disconnected, to speak to you, the constantly connected. That is why I hate Call Waiting. Click. Click. They always take that call and tell me goodbye. So I have Call Answering, New England Tel's voice mail system. It used to be hard to get away to a meeting. Now with electronic wizardry, it is as if one never left. I have two computers, one at work, one at home, and a laptop ordered so I can keyboard on a plane or a hotel room.

I was in Chicago last weekend and, without a keyboard, had an anxiety attack. I had to catch up on *U.S. News and World Report, Vanity Fair, GQ,* the *Boston Globe, New York Times, Perspectives, MT Monthly, The Latest Word, Journal of AAMT, Journal of AHIMA,* two novels, and *People* magazine. Imagine all of that on CD-ROM.

Between home and office, I have two computers, operate three digital dictation systems, two transcribers, and practice safe fax. Dial 1 if you know the party to whom you are speaking, dial 2 if you wish a Chinese interpreter, dial 3 to leave voice mail, and dial 4 if you do not have a touch-tone phone and are using a stupid rotary system. By the way, have you noticed how much more time it takes to telephone now?

I developed a head tremor, carpal tunnel syndrome, slight nystagmus on vertical gaze, and wear to bed, among other things, splints. I carry a little book with entry codes, passwords, and my PIN number. Just when I thought I had it under control, I have to get on a superhighway of information and master it. "Cyberspace—a wanderer on the electronic prairie," as one writer put it. It isn't enough that I am guilty about being overweight, guilty about not knowing enough about CompuServe, Delphi, Prodigy, E-mail, bulletin boards, emoticons, and snailmail. In school I had to learn Latin, Greek, French, Russian, and Polish and I can't master a smiley face using a colon, a dash, and a parenthesis.

We have come a long way from the time Jack Kennedy wooed America by his appearance on the debates with Nixon and his judicious use of television, to Bill Clinton wiring the White House for E-mail. All of us online, on call, on stage, and on board. Lexis/Nexis, Mosaic, Tlnet and a chance to cruise the records of the National Institutes of Health, the World Health Organization, the National Library of Medicine. Usenet, Relay Chat, Hytelnet, the Hairnet for the follicularly challenged, "World Wide Web," the Federal Register and the Congressional Record, the Electronic Access bill, the AHIMA BBS, hyperspace, and virtual shopping. There is a new language or jargon developing on the BBS circuit, and if you think PITA is a bread, wrong. It's a pain in the aspidistra.

And consider the ramifications of virtual anything and the etiquette of cybersex. Or is that netiquette? If one is alone, in a virtual reality romance, at what point does one say, "How was I?" And then at what point does one answer, "You were great, my darling!"

Put on those goggles and play golf, perform surgery, fly a plane, or travel the Chunnel. I am that creature, like many of you, a Colossus of Rhodes, one foot in medical transcription and one foot in ownership/management. If you think there is such a thing as balance anymore (an overworked female sort of a word, balance), think again. The stimulation of this business is so intense as to often preclude rest. And with it the righteous contempt for the appalling ignorance of people who are not connected to ANYTHING.

At age 16, my grandmother escaped Eastern Europe on a ship, all alone, carrying a pillowcase filled with salted fish, gold coins, and jewels. So I believe it was my family who originated the phrase "the smell of money." Grandmother had less trepidation coming to America than I have gingerly stumbling into the quicksand of limitless information.

Do I really want to communicate with 20 million people on the Net? I don't know about you folks, but I owe my **mother** a phone call. The work world and home are blurring together. Because the networks are out there, being a consumer means we **know** we have to use them.

I will spare you the dreadful similes associated with the information highway. I want to cheerfully park in the breakdown lane a moment.

There is something appealing about the cold beckoning screen, however, perhaps because of my sense of ultimate control or ultimate power, but who wields it, the machine or me? There is immense satisfaction in opening a file, a clean screen, not unlike the thrill of the bingo game. There are probably closet bingo players in this august body, though I readily admit to it. Mr. or Ms. Employer, put this question on your applications: Do you play bingo? Anyone who can play 27 cards, talk, eat, smoke, listen to the numbers, watch three or four television screens in the hall and do a triple bingo with two wild numbers makes a great transcriptionist.

MTs have such **focused** jobs. No calls, no calendars, no secretarial folderol, so every keystroke, every detail, takes on an exaggerated importance. Which often explains their violent attachment to their Lanier system or their VDI system or their transcriber or their computer. Their frustration and anguish when a report disappears on the system, poof! They look to managers and owners for direction in a computerized work world. They worry about having a job in the next ten years, just as we worry about having a product and in what permutation that product will be.

The literature is full of doctors who are at the ready, light pens in hand, trained in voice-activated dictation, or who have mastered the Olympus Endospeak or other softwares. My feeling is we still have enough bumblers in the business, punching in the wrong patient record numbers and the wrong report codes, to make the whole cycle good for a few years yet. Unless the whole form changes and we go from lengthy narrative summaries and operative notes to bursts of codes uttered by the physician or created by an interactive doc-screen configuration.

Transcription is, of course, intensely personal. As an MT in Sacramento told me in 1993, "I love my work. It is knowing the words and deliciously tasting them, chewing on them, and having them come out my fingers."

With more than 500 cable channels available in the near future, menus and options dazzling, tantalizing, videophone, home-based grocery shopping—will paper become obsolete? The merger of television, computers, and phones is yet to come. Will the smell of a new book overpower the sound of the modem connecting? Curling up with a you-know-what, will that become passe? Will the infotech workers become the drones, on a cradle-to-grave minimum wage journey not unlike McDonald's? Will the value of the transcribed medical record be distilled down because the meat of it will have become a menu-driven interchange between a doctor and computer? Who will control the Medinet—HCFA, JCAHO, AHIMA?

The office staff is delighted I am here. The hypercritical nitpicker is out of their files for four days. I read over their shoulders mercilessly. They ask me one question, I give them four corrections.

Transcriptionists really are the most conservative body on the face of the earth, with the possible exception of Polish Catholicism. They are very conservative when it comes to their actual labor and thought processes. I am a floor supervisor so I am working with the best of them and understand the frustration in being monitored by the hospital on the other end of the digital system. "You have been on the same 6-minute report for 20 minutes. We are watching your light."

I know how they feel when we are not consulted on headings being programmed into a system, for example. It is a very shaky feeling having a document uploaded immediately into a hospital mainframe.

What do I see in the future of the industry? There will be a shift from the lengthy narrative summary and operative report and consultation to a more standard dictation. This will change our requirements for transcriptionists and increase our markets in archiving and data retrieval.

There will be a proliferation in software such as Endospeak by Olympus and products such as Sudbury System's SmartType. Transcriptionists will be transcribing first, learning terminology later. Transcriptionists will still be medical language specialists but there will be more standardization of the language and of the format (thank God).

There will be more men in management and they will change how we deal with physicians. More likely the person in charge of transcription, the health information manager, will have an MBA and report to the vice president of finance.

This is not a sexist observation. Men dealing with men will have a major impact on this business. Many of you have read my criticisms of having parties and other incentives for physicians to do their job, i.e., complete the record, provide signatures. There will be a long-overdue demise to the philosophy of "Let's not disturb our doctors. They'll never change. Shut up and type."

There will be more training for doctors in how to dictate, not because it is the right thing to do or it would have been done long ago, but because it will cost money if it is done wrong.

In ten days I will be sitting in a garden at the Villa Medici in Florence. No phone. No computer. Not even a purse. Just antiquities, art, pasta, and vino. I am getting off this highway for a rest. Arrivederchi!

April 1994

The Tunakata
from Guatemala

The first time I saw that campus, it looked like the glittering set of Doctor Zhivago's country home in winter. I did not want to go there. I had a good job as transcription manager with IDS, Inc., but the Carroll Center in Newton, Massachusetts, needed a teacher for Beginning Medical Transcription, seven months, three times a week. My employer graciously allowed the flexible schedule, and on Valentine's Day 1994 we began.

Having no experience with the blind or handicapped, I made predictable errors. Soon, the eggs were teaching the chicken, and in the end it was I who was the student. I spent the first two weeks speaking too loudly and talking down to them. I pushed furniture around and tried to be too helpful. I knew enough not to pet the dogs or kiss them unless their harness was down, but I was jumpy and unsure of other doggy etiquette.

I had nightmares about the students' faces, their large unseeing eyes. I felt guilty because I was not blind. I felt guilty because I wanted to complain and whine, when, indeed, I was blessed because I could see. Stupidly, I said, "Don't try to do that without such-and-such a book, otherwise you are flying b-----, without a net." They set me straight. "Go ahead, say it, flying *blind*. We watch videos and we see our friends just like you." Then began the true education of Judith.

The winter was brutal. Boston broke a record for snowfall. Sidewalks were glassy. Huge snowbanks on the street by the bus stop made any foot travel hazardous. They never complained. The students mastered their computers, voice synthesizers and systems, and were forced to listen to me spelling and enunciating relentlessly. All the textbooks were available on tape, but the words were often mispronounced and never spelled. Of the six people, five lived on campus. They gave up their apartments and homes and lived in a dormitory, in class five days a week, eight hours a day. They endured winter, the lack of privacy, adjusting to a regimented series of mealtimes, and reading constantly, transcribing, and memorizing. They never complained.

One of my friends said that after childbirth she had no shame; there was no privacy in Labor and Delivery. For the medical transcription students, and for seven full months, they similarly gave up what private lives they had and became totally focused on the learning, and everything they did was scrutinized and judged. During our Round Table sessions, we listened to the SUM Program tapes, and I had all six sets of their transcripts in front of me. They did not have the luxury of reviewing their own work. This led to the usual repartee in such settings. "Creative transcription," I would say. "Close, but no cigar."

We had our usual student-at-work misfires. The patient with the last *minstrel* period and the wet *mop* (mount) test. Students were encouraged never to guess, rather to leave a blank. "A blank is an honorable thing," says Vera Pyle. "It means you don't know." Of course, they wanted to know what word they had put. In place of *tunica vaginalis*, a different word appeared. "What did I put?" A fair question. Reluctantly. "Tunakata." She said, "What is that?" "Sounds like Japanese catfood to me."

Thereafter I laughed harder than I ever had in my life. It was the kind of laughter that bubbles up and erupts in showers with no hope whatever of stifling. It was the kind of laughter that spread among us until the halls rocked. We were all left weak and panting. Administration wondered what was going on in the computer lab. I told them I would have to wear Depends to every session and went from there to the office with black mascara streaks all over my face. After that, errors became "tunakata." We also used "Oops." A generic sort of mistake, where no excuse is necessary.

We transcribed a case of a woman testing for STDs, including Chlamydia, Trichomonas, and Guatemala. Quite naturally, the Tunakata from Guatemala was born, much like the Girl from Ipanema. Gardnerella was the intended bull's-eye. Close, but no cigar.

I am going to miss this group. I am going to miss their tenacity in the face of illness and storms and the insurmountable gobbledygook that is the language of medicine spoken by physicians. I told them I don't want their love, but I would like their respect. Someday they are going to be transcribing and will be pitted against some faker or amateur. They will know they were trained the hard way, the best way, the complete way by a middle-aged fanatic who, though not a purist, was always demanding and tough and, at times, a raving lunatic.

They are going to remember that *sella turcica* is a Turkish saddle and understand the difference between *discrete* lymphadenopathy and my *discreet* affair with the milkman. They will understand the difference between an acronym and a homonym, who Dr. Gram was with his famous stain and Dr. Apgar and her famous scores.

They learned anatomy with the help of a real skeleton (not plastic) and a body model (real plastic). They know there is *Pap* and *pap*. They are thinking about the issues of premature babies, Do Not Resuscitate status, geriatric care muddles, and AIDS patients who require a cornucopia of free care. They know their bones, joints, and muscles, their mucus and mucous, and, oh God, they make me proud to have worked with them. They *are* medical language specialists.

They are taking the risk of their lives. They are willing to give up their income of SSI (Social Security). Their subsidized housing (25-30% of their income) would continue but not their Medicaid benefits. They want to work. I thought they received $1000 plus per month. Wrong. More like $650. No food stamps. Many of them have ended up with blackened faces in the backfire of some government program. In many cases, they might as well be making brooms in some sheltered workshop while their brains rot. Society says the goal is to mainstream, then holds back and says, no, not in my office.

So, if you are thinking about teaching and you are qualified, get involved. If you are an employer, hire a qualified medical transcriptionist as a trainee. If you can't hire, then provide an internship at least. You will get a lot more than the tax credit. Think about volunteering as a reader, especially if you know the correct pronunciation of medicalese. This is a computer age. Telecommuting may be a way of tapping a labor pool even more eager and hard-working than you had imagined.

Ginger Rogers did everything Fred Astaire did, but she did it backwards and wearing high heels. Now think about the blind, the handicapped, and take a step towards the future that includes them. They are just like us and dancing as fast as they can.

August 1994

I've Got a Secret

"Gentlemen: Please accept my resignation. I don't care to belong to any social organization that will accept me as a member." Groucho Marx to the Friars Club, published in *Groucho Phile*, 1976.

It was a beautiful hotel in Maine and a lovely spring AAMT symposium. Over 120 men and women were in that hall and I knew many of them. But not all of them. The chairperson of the event asked what she could have done to make it better. "List all the attendees and their business information and include it in your event folder of the day." "We can't do that," she said. "It would be a breach of confidentiality."

It was the same story in Washington, D.C., at the annual meeting of AAMT in 1992. "Post the name of the person you wish to see on the bulletin board and maybe they will see it and contact you." That was the official answer.

I got the same answer recently from my local chapter. The board of directors had voted and the membership list was not for distribution. "Some of the women think it is a breach of privacy," she said, rather huffily. So I decided to call around and ask a few chapter presidents their policy. Some said they never thought about it. Some said they

121

were never asked for one. Some said no membership list was readily available because it was a breach of privacy.

Middle age can be wonderful. The fire in the belly dies down or I take Maalox, the battles sort themselves out and people mellow. Some things that were so very important no longer are.

No longer the Young Turk I once was, I fork over my ever-increasing dues to AAMT and, in general, say little. Over 15 years of membership, the organization provided me with much more than I ever gave. I never was very political anyway. Shot my mouth off a lot, but the legacy is still there. That tiny chapter I helped found, nestled in the rolling hills of central Massachusetts, still clings to life. (Bay State, co-founded with Linda Simpson, CMT.)

The focus of our founders was education and networking. When Jackie Hagedorn came to town, speaking our lingo and said we were now part of something larger than any of us, created by us and for us, well, we just went wild. We could use a shot of Jackie right about now. Transcriptionists were never able to be a cohesive force and certainly last in that hospital hierarchy of the gods. Transcription companies were off site and out of sight. Telecommuting scattered the transcriptionists even more. AAMT was our chance to be with our own kind, learn, and network.

The education is wonderful. I think the speakers and information imparted are very exciting. The opportunity to see the slides or touch the pacemakers or view the magnetic resonance imaging is just as thrilling as it was more than a decade ago. The vendors are splendid and allow us to peruse the tools we need. Local chapter meetings, symposia, and the annual meetings are all worthwhile and I have many years of memories. So what is my grievance?

I want a list of the attendees, their names and their business affiliation provided to me routinely at every national meeting and every symposium. I want a membership list of my chapter provided to me annually. **I do not want to belong to a secret society.** I refuse to belong to a group which collectively does not wish it known they are a group and only the "officers" know who belongs.

The AAMT national office rents its membership lists and I am glad they do. I get interesting and germane advertising unless I refuse to allow my name to be used, which, of course, I don't. The national office makes a buck by renting the lists and I receive useful information related to my profession.

At that meeting in March it was evident what a collection of cliques we have become. Newcomers attend and no one pays much attention to them and they don't come back. Why not have an asterisk next to the name of the newcomer so people in the hall could make a special effort to say howdy and welcome? Professional groups and societies do this all the time. But an asterisk needs a list.

Why do I want a list? I wanted the list of chapter members at one point to write and telephone and ask if anyone needed work for a two-week period. Another time I wanted to know if anyone was considering a career change, as we had an opening in our office. Later I wanted to trade ideas with someone doing in-service education on confidentiality. At another time I wanted to know who had a visually-impaired transcriptionist on their staff so we could have a mutually beneficial discussion. Once I wanted to share my car with anyone wanting a ride to an out-of-state symposium, just to have some companionship; I could scroll down the membership list and see who lived nearby. No list. I drove alone. This tale is ridiculous in the telling, since the need is so obvious.

I always felt the local chapter was my sisterhood, my forged chain link of shared experience and knowledge. **I don't feel that way anymore.**

We are missing the boat here: Education and networking, the twin foundation of AAMT. Membership is not up; it is down. A shrinking number of people are now paying more money per person to support an enlarging national budget. And that loyal membership is aging. When I try to get people to join and I tell them the dues, they laugh at me. The hospital won't pay their dues. The company won't pay their dues. Everyone is *cutting* costs, not *increasing* them.

At a national meeting I am in a hall with over 600 people. If I do not recognize them, I don't know them. A list would help me to meet people in a rational, logical way. Someone I have read about, perhaps, who is using a certain computer system at their hospital. Someone whose writing I have long admired. Someone who has won an award, perhaps, and I read about it and want to congratulate them in person. Someone who works for a national company and I want to talk to them about that company and see if they are hiring. Someone who holds a similar position to mine in their company and might be willing to share information about quality analysis. Someone who has written about human resources tips on hiring transcriptionists. That is what the national meeting is about, isn't it? Education and networking. When I know who is there, I can put notes on the bulletin board.

People, this is a *business*. We have got to survive. No, we have to do more than survive; we must flourish and prosper. We need to keep the members we have. Everyone I ever met through AAMT was proud of their affiliation. We continually need new members. And it's not just their money we need. We need their youth, energy, freshness, and invigorating new ways of looking at things and doing things. We have become stale, even moribund.

We need people new to us, or people who perhaps strayed away from us, people with luminescent and cobweb-free minds. People just starting out and willing to belong, despite the restrictive and costly policy of student membership espoused by the AAMT national office in Modesto. People whose children are grown and have time and energy once again.

So where does all this talk about privacy and confidentiality and breaches thereof come from? **We have made ourselves so "private," we don't know who we are anymore.**

Our leaders are immersed in chasing non-issues of transcriptionist malpractice insurance, creating a task force for further research, fueling a blaze they are igniting themselves. There has never been a documented case of malpractice on the part of a transcriptionist in the history of the United States. This became a ridiculous priority and the House of Delegates let it happen.

The rules have changed. Members cannot just belong to local chapters; they must belong to national AAMT. This is a good and logical change. It is about time. Or is it too late? Will this be the deathknell of many small chapters, who have a sustained loyalty to each other and their chapter, and little to faraway national headquarters? By that logic, instead of having these members come to national, the chapter will cease to exist and the members will disperse. Instead of pumping in the blood to national, a local hemorrhage will occur. (Forgive me my little medical metaphor here.)

I hope that scenario is wrong. I've probably invested more time and money into AAMT than in my various marriages and degrees. I want a return on my investment. I want less fluff and harebrained non-issues and some basic business sense. Many of us are the loyal opposition, hanging on, clinging dearly to the professional organization.

Everyone loses if AAMT is diminished. American healthcare loses. The employers lose educated workers. The workers lose the education and we all go backwards. Or maybe we go en masse to AHIMA if their "open" membership passes. Or maybe MTIA will open membership to medical transcriptionists.

Or maybe we just disappear as a discrete entity. No one would miss us. We're not on any list.

September 1994

Glossary

AAMT (American Association for Medical Transcription), P. O. Box 576187, Modesto, CA 95357. Phone 209-551-0883, 800-982-2182. Fax 209-551-9317.

AHIMA (American Health Information Management Association), formerly AMRA (American Medical Record Association), 919 N. Michigan Avenue, Suite 1400, Chicago, IL 60611. Phone 312-787-2672. Fax 312-787-9793.

AMA (American Medical Association).

AMRA (American Medical Record Association), former name of AHIMA.

ART (Accredited Record Technician), an AHIMA credential.

CEC (Continuing Education Credit), earned by Certified Medical Transcriptionists to maintain certification.

CMT (Certified Medical Transcriptionist), an AAMT credential.

HCFA (Healthcare Financing Administration).

HIM (Health Information Management), formerly called *medical records management.*

HPI (Health Professions Institute).

JCAHO (Joint Commission on Accreditation of Healthcare Organizations).

MTIA (Medical Transcription Industry Alliance), P. O. Box 1491, Modesto, CA 95353. Phone 209-551-MTIA. Fax 209-551-0404.

MTs (medical transcriptionists).

PRD+ (an abbreviation expansion program), marketed by Productivity Software International, 211 East 43rd Street, Suite 2202, New York, NY 10017. Phone 212-818-1144. Fax 212-818-1197.

RRA (Registered Record Administrator), an AHIMA credential.

SUM Program (Systems Method Unit), a training program for medical transcriptionists developed and marketed by HPI.

The Author

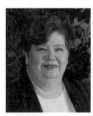

Judith Zielinski Marshall, a native Cleve-
lander, received B.A. and M.A. degrees in
History at Cleveland State University and
moved to Boston in 1976. She has over
twenty years of hospital transcription experience and is a former service owner. She
and her husband, Stuart, a retired Boston
University professor, live with their two golden retrievers,
Amber Rose and Angel.

Her first collection of essays, *Medicate Me*, was published in 1987 (Health Professions Institute, Modesto, Ca.).